Water Birth Unplugged

Proceedings of the
First International Water Birth Conference

Edited by
Beverley A. Lawrence Beech

D1334105

Books for Midwives Press
An imprint of Hochland & Hochland Limited

Published by Books for Midwives Press, 174a Ashley Road, Hale, Cheshire, WA15 9SF, England.

© 1996, Beverley Lawrence Beech

First edition.

ISBN 1-898507-53-8

British Library Cataloguing in Publication Data
A catalogue record for this book is available from the British Library

Cover illustration by Granville Rush, 'Happy Days', Broxted, Essex

Printed in Great Britain by Cromwell Press Ltd.

Contents

Part Seven: Water Birth Internationally

Part Eight: Water Birth - The Way Forward

Introduction by Sheila Kitzinger

Sheila Kitzinger is a social anthropologist and mother of five daughters. She is author of 24 books. The most recent include *'Ourselves as Mothers'*, *'The Year After Childbirth'*, *'Home Birth'*, *'Pregnancy and Childbirth'*, *'Birth Over 35'*, *'Freedom and Choice in Childbirth'* and *'The Experience of Childbirth'*. In 1982 she was awarded an MBE for her services in education for childbirth and parenting. Her faith in the natural ability of women to give birth has been a source of strength and guidance to women throughout the world. Sheila was one of the organizers of this conference.

In the Spring of 1995 1,500 midwives, doctors and mothers from countries all over the world crowded into the Wembley Conference Centre in London to share experiences and to learn about water birth. The International Water Birth Conference was organized by four women: Janet Balaskas of the Active Birth Movement, Beverley Lawrence Beech of the Association for Improvements in the Maternity Services, Jayn Ingrey of Splashdown Water Birth Services, and myself. It was a venture of faith, and we did it without sponsorship and with the deep conviction that it was vitally important for practitioners and researchers in water birth to get together to understand and to explore the effects of what is virtually an entirely new environment for birth.

The Water Birth Conference was arranged with three goals in mind: first that an international network of those working in water birth could be developed, because midwives often feel isolated and sometimes very threatened. At present many midwives, and the vast majority of obstetricians, have no experience of water birth, and in most hospitals where water births take place they are attended by only a few midwives who have developed specialist knowledge through seminars, reading and empirical learning. Moreover, even in hospitals where a birth pool is available, it may be little used, so that it is difficult for midwives to have confidence in their skills.

Another reason why this conference was important was to enable those who assist at water births, together with women who have experienced water birth, to focus on how birth can be a deeply satisfying experience for all those involved. When women who have used water in childbirth are asked to comment on the birth experience they almost invariably express positive feelings, and if they intend to have another baby, wish to give birth in water again. For anyone who has attended a labour when a woman is immersed in water the benefits are clear. There is mounting evidence that immersion in water relieves pain. A woman relaxes better, moves more easily, and is subjected to fewer interventions, such as frequent vaginal examinations, intrusive monitoring, perineal counterpressure, commanded pushing and prolonged breath-holding and episiotomy.

Moreover, there are significant general environmental changes associated with the introduction of birth pools in hospitals: dimmed lights, the practice of aromatherapy, and the sensitive use of touch and massage, while caregivers kneel on the floor or sit on a low stool, rather than standing over the woman in labour. All these mean that the woman is more likely to feel calm and unrushed, emotionally supported, among friends, and in control. Birth pools have brought a special quality to the environment of birth, helping midwives get back to their roots of working with women, and giving women power over the way they birth.

Anxiety is an intrusion in childbirth that is usually unrecorded and often undetected. Yet it can affect the thinking, actions and interaction of both the mother and her caregivers. It reduces the capacity to reason and leads to stressful relationships. At its most extreme it produces panic. It is relatively simple to record interventions that can be measured, but much more difficult to be aware of and to analyse the effects of anxiety on perception, behaviour and relationships. Anxiety may be one of the most dangerous elements to intrude on childbirth.

Searching questions must be asked about water birth. The conference provided a strong stimulus to research into the benefits and risks of water in labour and birth and served to create a new international network of those engaged in research. Researchers are asking such questions as:

- How safe is it?
- What are the potential risks?
- How effective is immersion in water as relief for pain and does it reduce the need for pain-relieving drugs?
- Does being in water reduce the need for operative deliveries?
- Has it any effect on the perineum, and the number of episiotomies that are performed and lacerations that occur?
- What are the postpartum outcomes for the baby and for the mother: what proportion of babies is admitted to the special care nursery, and does it have an effect on rates of postpartum haemorrhage and infection?
- How should midwives change their practice when helping women give birth in water instead of on land?
- Most important: how does water birth compare, in terms of safety for the baby, maintenance of the normal physiology of labour and birth, pain relief for the mother, and her satisfaction with the birth experience, with other ways in which labour is managed today, and with the invasive procedures that are accepted as normal practice, and that often go unquestioned because they are part of established hospital protocols and familiar routines?

Many techniques have been introduced into obstetrics since the 1970s which have been inadequately researched, which have been imposed on women, and which have radically altered the environment of birth.

Continuous electronic fetal monitoring, for example, has become an established and unquestioned procedure in hospitals all over the world. Since its widespread acceptance, research has revealed that it is of no benefit to mothers and babies. Yet women are still harpooned to monitors, and caregivers continue to place confidence in monitor printouts which have no significance for birth outcomes, and which they are frequently unable to interpret accurately. While using the language of choice, hospitals offer a primarily electronic environment for birth in which the woman is expected to be a passive and obedient patient.

In a similar way, there have been no randomized controlled trials of the side-effects of epidural anaesthesia. Epidurals are promoted to pregnant women as safe and without harmful side-effects, though there is evidence that it may be associated with a long-term backache and headache. An epidural also raises the mother's temperature during birth. We know that the temperature of the fetus is higher than the mothers, and that if she is pyrexic the baby is put at risk. This is one of the concerns that has been expressed, quite rightly, when women are immersed in hot water in a birth pool. The remedy is simple and the water is cooled to body temperature by adding cold water. Yet though this is a perceived risk with water birth, and one which has achieved headlines in the British press, similar publicity has never been given to the less easily controlled effects of fever with epidural anaesthesia.

We must not make the mistakes that have been made in obstetrics when, for example, wholesale induction of labour and the immobilization and tethering of women to intravenous drip stands became standard practice without adequate investigation; when routine ultrasound scans throughout pregnancy came to be accepted as good practice without any evidence; when a pregnant woman with sugar in her urine and blood was labelled as having a disease called 'gestational diabetes', and one with reduced levels of haemoglobin in late pregnancy was labelled as 'anaemic', both of which diagnoses resulted in anxiety-arousing treatments and investigations for what has been revealed as a normal condition. We advocate vigorous evaluation of and multicentre international research into the physical, social and psychological effects of the use of birth pools.

Data obtained from 19,000 water births that have taken place in different countries was presented at the conference and indicate that the use of water is associated with fewer forceps deliveries and Caesarean sections and reduces the chances of other interventions in childbirth.

Detailed statistical analysis of case records of water births in Vienna, Malta and London reveals that water reduces the need for pain-relieving drugs, together with the risks that come with all anaesthesia; a woman's uterus is more likely to function effectively in labour without requiring drugs to stimulate activity; and she is more likely to have an intact perineum, and significantly less likely to have an episiotomy or third degree tear, when she gives birth in water. There is no evidence that water birth is dangerous for babies. In fact, in some studies fewer babies needed to be resuscitated or go to the intensive care nursery after they had been born in water.

The first International Water Birth Conference was unique in drawing together researchers, midwives, obstetricians, paediatricians and neonatalogists, general practitioners, birth educators, obstetric physiotherapists, sociologists and parents with the experience of water birth from nineteen countries, including places as far apart as Australia, the Russian Federation, the United States, Europe, both East and West, Japan, South America and Africa. This selection of papers from the Conference is an indication of how they shared their knowledge and laid the foundations for future research.

Opening Address by Baroness Cumberlege

Baroness Cumberlege was appointed Under-Secretary of State for Health in 1992 and from 1981-88 was Chairman of South West Thames Regional Health Authority and a Council Member of the United Kingdom Central Council for Nursing, Midwifery and Health Visiting from 1989-92. In 1992 she was appointed Chair of the Department of Health's Expert Maternity Group. This group was charged with responding to the proposals made by the Parliamentary Health Select Committee (The Winterton Report) and in August 1993 published *Changing Childbirth*, a review of the maternity services designed to encourage change in the quality and focus of maternity care in England and Wales. She is married to a farmer and has three sons.

When you become a Minister you are always very conscious of how the urgent always pushes out the important, and it's very easy to spend the whole of your life reacting to events, responding to the media, replying to Parliamentary debates, submissions from officials, and you have to make up your own mind, have I got a personal agenda, what do I want to achieve?

In 1987, I went to talk to a very large gathering of health visitors, and in that talk I just remarked how very sad I was. How to me, birth had lost its magic and its mystery. How it had really been highjacked by high tech medicine. That throwaway remark generated thunderous applause, and I thought, this is very interesting, I really have touched a nerve. I must look more carefully into it. That's when I started to read a lot of articles by Sheila Kitzinger, and other people, and realized what a miserable experience childbirth can be for so many women.

In 1991, just before I had been made a Minister, the Social Services Select Committee of the Houses of Parliament undertook an Enquiry into maternity services, commonly called the Winterton Report. Having read that, I agreed with so much of it and I was very grateful to that Committee of Parliament, who had talked to a lot of women, who challenged a lot of the current traditional thinking and practice, and who broke some of the windows that needed breaking.

In a way it was quite surprising that they decided to look at the maternity services, because if you look at it statistically it is a huge success. Infant mortality has improved dramatically over the last ten years, a reduction of 40 per cent - that's equivalent to 2000 fewer deaths per year, a huge achievement.

I was looking only this week at the Office of Population Censuses and Surveys published figures for 1992, the latest ones produced, and, again, our figures are lower than they have ever been. So in this respect, maternity services have been a great success. Once a Committee of Parliament produces a Report the Government has to respond. I thought this is just great, this gives me the opportunity I want in order to make some changes.

So, we set up a team to respond to the Winterton Report, a team of eight, and I chaired it. Out of those eight, four were consumers, four were professionals, and this is one of the very first committees that the Government has ever produced with 50 per cent consumers or, with me, over 50 per cent.

So, it was a radical change, but I have to say that we did rely very heavily on our professionals in the team, one of whom was Professor Lesley Page, who will be talking to you tomorrow. From the consumers, we had the President of the National Childbirth Trust, a voluntary organization in our country; a management consultant; somebody who had been very active in the Asian Mother and Baby Campaign; and a journalist on the *Sunday Times*, who was expecting twins at the time.

So we got together, and it was a really difficult subject to think about. How did we want to change it? What did we want to see, say, in five years time? What would maternity services look like if we could have the ideal?

We decided on five principles.

- First of all that it should be a woman-focused service. We wanted to put the woman back into the driving seat. It was no good having the best services in the world if they were not accessible.

- We said they ought to be easily accessible.

- We wanted services to be responsive but not just responsive, also effective.

- We wanted to ensure that women were involved with the planning of their services, and that they could have an input early on.

- We also recognized, as taxpayers, with a publicly funded NHS, it was absolutely essential that we made the best use of resources.

So that was really our ideal, and then we went back and we looked at the people who used the services. We talked to hundreds of women during the nine months that we undertook the report. We were very conscious that women who used maternity services are quite different from other client groups within the NHS. To begin with, they are pretty fit and well, they are alert, they even go into training for the great event. They are well informed, they're knowledgeable, demanding, and although we recognized that every single woman is different, we also appreciated that as a group they had different aspirations from other people using the National Health Service, and were so different from those using the services 40 years ago. If you look back to the 1950s I think it was James Thurber who said that 'a woman's place is in the wrong'. Well a woman's place in the 1950s was certainly in the home, and for those who did do work it was for low pay, had low status, and was an undemanding job.

Today it is different. Today there are women who are breaking the glass ceilings, women who are getting to the top, women in the media, barristers, bankers, journalists, my goodness, even priests! Women in positions of authority, really changing society, in control of their lives; and not only their lives but often as managers of other people's lives. They are asking questions: 'we keep appointments in our businesses, why doesn't the NHS?'

When you look at the age of women having their first babies the average is 28. So, they are much more mature, confident, women. But you will say to me: 'that is only a tiny minority of women who are in these positions', and of course you are right. Many, many more are struggling on low incomes, they are less articulate, and that is why it is so important that we listen to them more carefully, because they find it more difficult to express their views. We do no favours to them if we remove responsibility at the beginning, during pregnancy and labour and then expect them to take responsibility for the new life which they have spawned.

When talking to the women, we asked what they themselves wanted, and in fact were amazed at how very, very, modest women's demands are. They want just three things:

- choice
- continuity
- control

They wanted a choice of professional: midwife, GP, obstetrician, shared care, and we thought it was absolutely right that they should have that choice. After all, this is a huge event in one's life. We choose our friends, how much more important to choose our professional friend, whom we can trust and know will be sympathetic.

They wanted choice in the place of birth: high-tech, midwifery led or GP led care, birth at home, or in hospital. We conducted a Mori poll, and found that three-quarters of the women questioned said that they were given no choice. When given a choice we found dramatic changes. In part of London, two years ago, two per cent of women had home births, today it is up to 12 per cent. I think that does show that if you give people choice they will exercise it.

But of course giving choice requires good information, and one of the things that we were very conscious of was how difficult it is to put over unbiased information. Our Report comes in two halves; the second half, which is separately bound, highlights good practice in information giving.

We also had a lot of discussion on safety, and we were conscious that over the years safety has been an excuse for a certain style of care of birth, and that once you get into interventions that leads onto more interventions and so on.

We felt that over the years, we had almost disabled women. We had reduced their confidence - the instincts they have about their own bodies.

We recognized that safety was part of the greater picture, a factor but not the sole factor. It was important in order to exercise choice, women had unbiased information, and I do congratulate those who are trying to get through this problem. We always acknowledge that safety has to remain the foundation of good maternity care. After all, every woman wants a safe delivery, a healthy baby and to be healthy herself.

Now part of this picture, part of the choice and part of safety is the question of water births. How does this fit into the picture, into the general context?. We very much welcome this conference today, which seeks to widen the debate, not only within the United Kingdom, but internationally.

Given the information, we believe it is right that women should choose the method that they feel will help them most. But it is also right that those methods should be evaluated, and I really am delighted that shortly Fiona Alderdice from the National Perinatal Epidemiology Unit, Oxford, will be publishing details of her recent study (Alderdice, 1995). We have also commissioned work by the Institute of Child Health, because we recognize that we need quite a number of studies to build up the whole picture. We look forward to their results at the end of the year.

In the Department of Health we have been supporting both these projects, through funding, and we are taking an active interest in other research worldwide. For we do want women to have the very best information, and the best evaluation before reaching their decisions.

After the question of choice, we recognize that women also want continuity, and wherever we went we heard this phrase: 'All I wanted was a familiar face'. We have instances of women telling us how they were delivered, not even knowing the people in the room. One saying: 'there was this strange man in the corner, I never knew who he was'.

Our journalist, who was having twins, saw 38 health professionals during the course of her antenatal period and the birth. We recognize that that is not good care, and it is often those at the most risk who actually get less continuity and who need it most.

We also felt that it was very important that midwives should be community based, that they should be not only in the community but of the community, recognized and known. When we looked at the question of control, we also recognized again the question of being fully informed. How can you be fully informed if you are uncertain about what is going on, what the options are, how to go forward? One of the things we found was in some areas, where women were holding their own notes, that these really gave them a bit more confidence, and that is something we recommend.

Now, looking to five years time how would we recognize *Changing Childbirth*, if introduced? We tried to picture it and identify indicators of success.

The first was that there should be a named midwife. We felt that was really important, in terms of continuity and it is part of the Patient's Charter that the midwife should be the lead professional in about 30 per cent of women being delivered, and I know now in places like Castlefields, a GP fundholding practice, direct access is always to the midwife. The GP does not get involved unless the woman wants it, or unless she needs him because she is ill.

We also felt that every woman should know her lead professional. Most women know their GP and midwife, but not all know the obstetrician. In fact, where we have run some pilot schemes we are finding that for instance at Kings, 96 per cent of those on the scheme do know the person who delivers them. We felt that was very important. We wanted midwives to have access to maternity beds, because that would give them some resource that they needed, and we felt it was very important to review antenatal care.

We also wanted to ensure that ambulancemen, paramedics, were well trained in case of emergencies. And lastly, very important, we wanted women to be well informed.

So, what has happened since we produced our Report? Well, it has been very warmly received, and a lot of credit goes to the Royal College of Midwives, and others, especially the voluntary groups: The National Childbirth Trust, the Association for Improvements in the Maternity Services and the Maternity Alliance, who gave us a huge amount of support.

The Report went out for consultation, and it was accepted by the Government as policy in January 1994. Once we got the go-ahead, we geared up the National Health Service to put it into practice, and we really believe that things are now beginning to happen working through Regional Health Authorities, and through the contracting mechanism.

We set up a national advisory group, of people from the Royal Colleges, professionals, and consumers, to keep a watching brief, but particularly to look at education and training.

We set up an implementation team, a small group with a full time Director, Kate Jackson, who is spreading good practice and is a wonderful resource for those people who want information and advice. We set up an evaluation programme because we recognized that it was really important to see the impact of what we were trying to do. We have also secured the future of the National Perinatal Epidemiology Unit, which is an enormously important organization giving accurate and well researched information to those who seek it, professionals and, we hope, increasingly women themselves, and I would like to congratulate them on the second edition of that all important book *Effective Care in Pregnancy and Childbirth*. We have also built this into the strategy for research. We have included a midwife on that team, to ensure that research for midwifery services gets a high profile, and we have included a midwife on the advisory group.

Now, I am very conscious that when you are trying to introduce something you cannot do it from top down, it has to be bottom up. To have people wanting to make the changes, and one of the huge forces for change are the women in this country. We are very lucky, for we have the Patient's Charter which sets out people's rights and standards and tells them what they can expect from the National Health Service. We have built on this, and we have been the first group to produce our own Charter for a specific service - this is the Maternity Charter. I really hope that women are using it, and professionals are aware of it and try to meet its rights and standards.

Rights and Standards permeate the whole philosophy of *Changing Childbirth*. The question of rights to see records and to keep them with you. Rights for fuller information of what is available. Choices: home, hospital, high tech, low tech, which professional you want. Questions about the named professional, that is a right; standards set for an appointment for antenatal clinics, 30 minutes, and I have to say that when I talk to women they can't believe we have set that standard. So, clearly, we are not meeting it.

Advice, respect, access. The Charter commits the NHS to showing consideration for privacy, dignity, cultural and religious beliefs. It is a powerful tool, and we very much hope that people will use it.

We have also taken other steps - the Royal College of Midwives and the Department of Health's visiting scholarship. Somebody who is concentrating on *Changing Childbirth* in an academic way.

We are producing videos for women, videos for professionals to help them give unbiased information. We are trying to support professionals through the *Changing Childbirth* Implementation Team, and also we have set up, last year, 14 pilot projects which we have funded. Now those pilot projects are across the country and we are asking for bids soon for this coming year. We will be putting one million pounds into new schemes.

So, we believe that we have made a start. We do not, in any way, underestimate the difficulties. It is a very, very, challenging programme. Its concepts aren't easy. I do accept that, and I do accept that the Devil is in the detail, but I am encouraged by the countless of thousands of health professionals, obstetricians, particularly midwives, and some GPs, up and down the country who recognize their time has come to deliver the highest quality care.

This is a moment of huge opportunity, this is a moment of professional fulfilment for midwives and doctors, and a time of enormous fulfilment for the women in their care. I am convinced that in five years time *Changing Childbirth* will have become a reality, and this Report can take its place on the shelf of history.

Reference

Alderdice, F., Renfrew, M. et al. (1995). 'Labour and birth in water in England and Wales: Survey report'. *British Journal of Midwifery,* Vol. 3, No.7, pp.375-382.

PART ONE

Why a Water Birth?

CHAPTER ONE

Birth in the 21st Century: Where are we Going?

Marsden Wagner completed his training in Medicine, Paediatrics, Neonatology, Public Health and Perinatal Epidemiology at the University of California at Los Angeles. After several years paediatric practice, teaching and research at UCLA he became Co-ordinator of Maternal and Child Health for the California State Department of Public Health. In 1971 he became the Director of the UCLA University of Copenhagen Health Service Research Centre based in Denmark. In 1978 he became the Director of Maternal and Child Health for the European Region of the World Health Organisation, based in Copenhagen, and responsible for consulting in 32 countries. He is a single father of four children. He has written over 80 publications including five books.

I will begin with an apology, because I am a man. That means I am an outsider at birth. I don't care if he is a Professor of Obstetrics, a man is an outsider at birth, so keep that in mind when I speak to you.

I worked at the World Health Organisation for 15 years and I want to talk a little bit about where birth is going and how water birth fits in.

Water birth, like home birth, is really symbolic of the non-orthodox, non-obstetric approach to birth; both of these phenomena use a social model rather than a medical model of birth, and there is a worldwide struggle going on between those two approaches.

I have just finished a paper called, 'The Global Witch Hunt' (Wagner, 1995) in which I review 20 court cases that I have been involved in. These court cases have been in the United States, Canada, Austria, Italy, Australia, New Zealand, Sweden, the United Kingdom, France and Germany. They most commonly involve midwives, because midwives are in the middle, between the medical and social models. They're very vulnerable standing in that spot. Some cases have involved doctors who have used some of the approaches, like water birth. If you use these kind of approaches, even if you are a doctor, you are vulnerable.

This century has really seen the takeover of birth by the obstetric profession. I am going to talk about the obstetric professional, and not about individual obstetricians who, of course, vary. The obstetric profession has fought hard and has succeeded in controlling birth.

In Spain, all midwifery schools have been closed. In France, last year, they passed a new law. They gave every Frenchwoman the right to demand an epidural, and I will talk later about the safety of epidurals. In Germany, a paper was published in the German Obstetrical Society Journal, using a lot of nonsensical 'science', in an attempt to prove that homebirth was dangerous. The German obstetricians demanded that the Government pass new laws to protect the fetus from the dangerous women.

Moving the birth to the hospital was part of the takeover because women wanted the birth in their territory, but now obstetrics has succeeded with hospitalizing almost everyone, to control birth and control women through technology. That's why I published a book last year called *Pursuing the Birth Machine* (Wagner, 1994) where I talk about these two approaches and all the new technology.

Nearly all these newer birth technologies have been inadequately scientifically evaluated. For example, while still in the WHO, we wrote a letter to the Governments in the European Region, urging them to reconsider policies on routine scanning of all pregnant women with ultrasound because new research – very good randomized controlled trials – showed that there is no benefit to scanning all women. In addition, other trials showed that, in fact, scanning during pregnancy may cause intrauterine growth retardation. When that letter went out to the Governments, you can't imagine the angry response against the WHO from the medical establishment, and in some cases the public health establishment in the European Region.

Now, there's an epidural epidemic in Europe. Yesterday, in Birmingham, I asked a room full of midwives about epidural use in their hospitals, and nearly every one of them said that their hospital was involved with over 50 per cent epidurals. Birthing women are being told that having an epidural is safe. While millions of women have been given epidurals, less than 600 have ever participated in a randomized trial as to the effectiveness and risks of this procedure. It is inadequately evaluated. Is it safe?

- There are 4–10 times as many forceps or vacuum interventions if you have an epidural;
- twice as many caesareans if you have an epidural;
- you are at risk of respiratory paralysis (you stop breathing);
- there is a ten per cent risk that the fetal heart will slow way down from lack of oxygen because the woman's blood pressure falls;
- the woman is at risk of severe chronic backache, etc. (American College of Obstetricians and Gynaecologists, 1995).

yet women are told that an epidural is safe and glorious.

Active management of labour is the quintessential example of the medicalization of birth. Obstetricians do too many caesarean sections so they come up with another technology to try to put the lid on this technology. They come up with aggressive, invasive procedures in order to try to stop doing so many caesareans. Of all the things that go on in active management, if you look at the science, the artificial rupture of the membranes does not lower the caesarean rates, the use of oxytocin doesn't lower the caesarean rates, the one thing that does is the continuous assistance of a midwife throughout labour. That is the only thing in active management that has been shown scientifically to reduce caesarean rates, and yet when people replicate active management elsewhere they don't even include that continuous midwifery element in their so-called active management.

> 'Many Western doctors hold the belief that we can improve everything, even natural childbirth to a healthy woman. This philosophy is the philosophy of people who think it deplorable that they were not consulted at the creation of Eve because they would have done a better job'. (Kloosterman, 1994)

I've watched water birth around the globe. I think probably my most profound experience was in the former Soviet Union. I spent a week on the Black Sea with Igor Tjarkovsky and a group of midwives and expecting families with sea birth. It was a profound experience, and I came away with an enormous admiration for those midwives and those families.

Water birth like homebirth is controversial. Why? Because the obstetricians are out of control. It's that simple. The water helps the woman, but it sure doesn't help the birth attendant. It's the opposite of the lithotomy position, which helps the birth attendant, but doesn't help the woman. With water birth, the birth attendant has many dilemmas, do I roll up my sleeves, do I get in the pool, do I take my clothes off, what do I do here?. You can't really attend a water birth and keep your sophisticated control and dignity.

There is good evidence that the childbearing pendulum is beginning to swing away from the medicalization and towards a more social model of birth. I think the next century will see a continuing erosion of obstetrical control. Birth will be gradually, but inexorably, returned to the woman. Midwives will no longer be 'with-doctor', midwives will be 'with-woman'. I think the British report 'Changing Childbirth' (Department of Health, 1993) is a wonderful example of the pendulum starting to swing. You'll be glad to know that they are reopening the midwife's school in Spain. You'll be glad to know that in Germany, as a result of all of this nonsense trying to outlaw homebirths, the midwives and the women's groups, and a few doctors and others, are getting organized. They are networking, and things are really starting to happen in Germany. Almost all of Canada now has finally legalized midwifery. They have a new midwifery law in New Zealand that is really strengthening midwifery. There is a midwifery renaissance around the globe. This is part of a bigger renaissance of women taking control over their own reproduction and bodies, and a general greater appreciation of the importance of women's health. Water birth is a piece of all of that, a very important symbolic piece of all of that.

I think we can be encouraged, the struggle is not over, we are going to go forward with love and with joy.

References

American College of Obstetricians and Gynaecologists (1995). 'Fetal heart rate patterns', *Technical Bulletin* 207, July.

Department of Health (1993). *Changing Childbirth, Report of the Expert Maternity Group*. Chaired by Baroness Cumberlege. London: HMSO.

Kloosterman, G. (1994). Paper presented in Barcelona at Perinatal Conference.

Wagner, M. (1994). *Pursuing the Birth Machine: The Search for Appropriate Birth Technology*. Sydney, Australia: ACE Graphics.

Wagner, M. (1995). 'A global witch-hunt', *The Lancet,* 346, pp.1020–22.

CHAPTER TWO

Why do Women want a Birth Pool?

Janet Balaskas is the director of the Active Birth Centre and a mother, childbirth educator and activist, who founded the Active Birth Movement in 1981. She is best known for empowering mothers to step off the delivery bed and reclaim freedom and control of their own births. She has been involved with water birth since 1987 when her husband Keith Brainin invented a portable birth pool system which would be used in any suitable birthing environment. The Active Birth Centre now runs a nationwide pool hire company and has supplied 125 hospitals with installed birth pools. This brings them into contact with a multicentred source of evaluative experience, research and information. Janet's workshops on water birth are highly regarded internationally. She is co-author of *Water Birth* with Yehudi Gordon as well as many other titles. Janet is one of the organizers of the conference.

I am speaking today on behalf of the millions of women like myself who would prefer to give birth without medical intervention, unless there is difficulty or a complication. Of course, we appreciate the help of doctors when we need it, but we expect a healthy pregnancy, more often than not, to be followed by an uncomplicated birth. It is in this context that we might think of using a birth pool.

My work as a childbirth educator is concerned with the empowerment of women during pregnancy, in preparation for birth and motherhood. Most of the mothers I work with approach me with a desire to give birth naturally. At first, they are usually apprehensive; somewhat daunted by the medical surveillance recommended by their doctors. Their confidence in their own potential to give birth has been undermined throughout their lives by the cultural attitudes they have grown up with. The main emphasis of the antenatal care they are receiving is screening for possible problems or pathology.

I take advantage of the remaining months of the pregnancy to increase their awareness of the miracle taking place in their bodies. I encourage them to think of giving birth as an exhilarating challenge, a powerful act of creation for which their bodies are perfectly made. I offer them an alternative to the prevailing attitude that a normal pregnancy is a potential illness, fraught with risks and dangers, needing the supervision of an obstetrician.

In my groups they meet other pregnant women at various stages of pregnancy. They discover new options and learn directly about the birth experiences of mothers returning to visit with their newborn babies soon after the birth. They soon learn that birth can be one of the most rewarding experiences a woman can have, the fruition of her sexuality and highlight of her family life. They, too, begin to look forward to sharing such an experience with their partner, welcoming their baby in a spirit of love and celebration.

However, in looking for an alternative to an obstetric delivery, most women are not thinking primarily of themselves. Their main concern is the quality of the birth experience for the baby. Women today are aware that to be born is a monumental and awesome experience. Like dying, it is sacred in a very special way. As mothers, women feel that they are responsible for bringing new life into the world. They want their babies to be safe and to be born in a gentle and loving way, without unnecessary trauma or violence.

This is why, in the first instance, they want to avoid the routine use of powerful drugs, chemicals and metal instruments wherever possible and it is the main reason why they are attracted to exploring the help of water in labour and also, sometimes for birth. In its essence, the philosophy of water birth is a practical development of the ideas of Frederick Leboyer, who first drew the world's attention to the quality of the birth and its importance to the baby, as well as the psychologists who led us to understand the relevance of our intrauterine and birth experiences to our emotional wellbeing throughout our lives.

To place water birth in context it is necessary first to look briefly at the historical and cultural background to this phenomenon. European women first lost touch with their power as birth givers when male barber physicians took over from midwives in the 17th Century. At this time women began to be on their backs for birth and forceps were invented. From these roots the obstetric management of childbirth developed. Obstetric procedures such as the use of forceps necessitated women lying on their backs. The supine position became the prevalent posture for birth and women became passive patients rather than active birth-givers.

With the increasing trend towards hospitalization and medicalized maternity units, the invention of anaesthesia and the availability of the modern caesarean section and other birth technology, birth became overwhelmed by obstetrics. This movement reached its peak by the 1970s, by which time the normal physiology of birth had been more or less totally eradicated and forgotten.

A recent version of the same tradition can still be seen today in most large modern hospital maternity units where uncomplicated, so called 'normal births' are taking place in an obstetric context. Here the idea is to control and monitor the birth – to do better than nature. This sort of birth is still endured today by far too many women – most of whom are unaware that there are other options.

Not only is the mother's power and pleasure usurped and the baby put at risk by such routines as enforced use of the reclining position, or continuous electronic fetal heart monitoring, but the baby may then be unnecessarily assaulted in the first minutes of life by premature clamping and cutting of the umbilical cord, unnecessary suctioning of the air passages and separation from the warmth and comfort of the mother's arms.

I don't have time to go into greater detail, it is clear that this approach to birth represents one of the most disastrous misunderstandings to happen in the name of science – one which has overlooked the fact that birth is an instinctive physiological process which is regulated by hormones produced by the mother herself. The hormonal flow in labour depends on her emotional state, which in turn is affected by how she is treated and the atmosphere in the birthing room.

Throughout the 1900s, women have been increasingly rebelling against the domination of birth by obstetrics and developing a worldwide counter-revolution, broadly known as the childbirth movement.

In 1982, in protest against such an approach to birth at my local hospital in North London, I joined with pregnant women, colleagues and midwives to form the Active Birth Movement. In that year we hosted two international conferences in this very hall as well as the Birth Rights Rally. This was a demonstration in the streets of London in which more than 5,000 women, supported by midwives, took action and refused to lie down and take it any longer. We were proclaiming publicly that Active Birth was here to stay. We can thank the pioneering mothers, who, in those early days, flew in the face of the doctor's dictate, to give birth on their own two feet. The positive outcomes of these births, the alert and untraumatized condition of these babies, made a deep impression on doctors and midwives who were used to seeing flat, 'Pethidined' babies.

Thirteen years on, Active Birth is far more widely accepted and it is now common for women throughout the United Kingdom to be encouraged to be mobile in labour. Greater freedom and more choice in childbirth are the basis of a new trend towards a more humane way of giving birth and welcoming the newborn into the world.

Both midwifery training and the recent recommendations of the Health Authority are supportive to developing a 'woman-centred' maternity care as we approach the year 2000.

We now need to ask questions such as:

- how can we create the best conditions for a physiological birth; and,
- how can we encourage the instinctive behaviour of mothers in labour?

A birth pool can play a very useful role in finding the answers to such questions. Unlike obstetrics, a water birth essentially facilitates the process of birth.

On one level, a birth pool represents a sanctuary from the menace of obstetric routines. Once the mother enters the protective womb-like space of the pool, it becomes much more difficult to disturb her. As she sinks into the warm water, her body becomes her own territory. Only with her willing cooperation and consent, can her attendants get close to her.

The presence of a birth pool, especially in a hospital, has an almost magical power to transform the birthing environment into something quite different from the clinical rooms designed for an obstetric birth.

When filled with warm water, a birthing pool positively invites the mother to relax. There is no delivery bed in sight. Technology takes a low profile, so that the usual atmosphere of fear and danger is eradicated.

The expectations of what is going to happen in a pool room are radically different from what we are used to in a hospital. The presence of a pool indicates there has been a deliberate attempt to induce feelings of confidence and relaxation in the mother. This makes the hospital environment far more attractive to mothers who are aiming to give birth physiologically, and would also like the security of obstetric support at close hand.

When we introduce a birth pool, it means creating an environment for the birth which I would call 'hormone enhancing'. A room in which the lights can be dimmed, there is a peaceful, calm, quiet atmosphere and a feeling of tremendous respect for the mother's need for privacy, along with the kind of support she, as an individual will need.

The crucial component in this environment is the motherly presence of a midwife whom the woman already knows and trusts. Ideally the mother and midwife will have had an opportunity to form a relationship prior to the birth and the prenatal care will have been the responsibility of the midwife or team of midwives attending the birth. It is important that the midwife is comfortable with water and has a non-interventionist approach to birth. A quality of protective emotional support and trust in the birthing mother's power, on the part of the midwife, is a natural accompaniment to the presence of a birth pool. Such a midwife is willing to re-evaluate her practise, to try the 'hands off' approach that is most appropriate to the use of a birth pool, knowing when it is really necessary to intervene.

Many midwives have told me that working with water has helped them to 'unlearn' old routine habits and to discover new ways of guiding the mother through labour. This is the kind of midwifery that women need and want for a physiological birth, whether in or outside a birth pool.

In parts of the United Kingdom there is an increase in the number of women giving birth at home, as awareness of this option grows. Prejudice against home births is being challenged and positively supported by the midwifery organizations as well as the health authorities and numerous consumer groups.

As an alternative to hospital water birth, many women prefer to hire a portable pool and set it up in the familiarity and comfort of their own home. Here the conditions for a natural birth are optimal and the power of water to enhance the progress of labour is profound.

The pool is prepared so that the water is comfortably warm, close to the mother's own body temperature and deep enough to cover her belly when kneeling. The mother usually enters the pool about half way through her labour. While there are some women who do not enjoy being in water in labour or find it disappointing, entering the warm water is an absolutely marvellous experience for most women. The first thing the mother feels is a sense of unimaginable comfort and relief as the water supports her body.

Water is a feminine element – like the ocean, it is the mother of all creation. Its presence creates a feminine atmosphere in the birthing room. Its buoyant quality carries the body's weight, so that it becomes much easier to change positions, for example to squat without support and to move freely.

It is a feeling of being physically liberated, something like the freedom to move which we experience when we play in warm water in a swimming pool or in the ocean. The soft, wet, sensuous caress of the water on the mother's skin reminds her that her labouring body is beautiful, powerful and sensual.

It helps her to perceive her birth giving as sexual, as a part of the loving relationship in which her baby was conceived. It makes it easier for her to lose her inhibitions to access the primordial sexual energy of her birth-giving power.

Being in warm water allows a deep and profound relaxation, as the world outside the rim of the pool recedes and a change of consciousness can occur. Mental control and inhibition give way to unthinking instinctual behaviour. The mother's body opens at its deepest centre preparing to release her baby in the orgasm of birth.

Birth giving is involuntary. It just happens, when we can let go and completely relax. Modern women sometimes find this letting go very difficult, so for them a birth pool can be a very effective way to facilitate this release.

As a mother of four myself and a childbirth educator with more than 15 years experience, I have tried every method going since Erna Wright's breathing techniques. I find immersion in warm water to be the most powerful and simplest way to encourage deep relaxation in labour.

Many positive effects of water immersion in labour have been observed. So, by way of an introduction, I will briefly explore these topics without going into detail. Most women think first of using a birth pool for pain relief. Water has the power to alter a woman's perception of pain – to help her to accept the intensity of the sensations she is experiencing, without needing to resort to other forms of pain relief. While many think that water immersion increases the secretion of 'endorphins' – our body's natural pain killers – in fact it appears that endorphin levels are reduced in a birth pool, indicating that pain levels are lower. While a birth pool doesn't usually take away all the pain, it can help to make it much less overwhelming, so that the mother feels that she is in control. This can make that marginal difference which results in the mother being able to manage the pain herself without recourse to analgesics.

Other possible benefits are as follows:

*   Faster, more efficient dilation, resulting in a shorter labour. This can lead us to assume that under these relaxed conditions the mother's brain produces greater levels of oxytocin – the hormone which stimulates uterine contractions – which Michel Odent calls the 'hormone of love'.
*   A lowering of blood pressure has been noted.
*   The buoyant effect makes water an excellent helper for disabled or obese women.
*   The humid atmosphere helps asthma sufferers.
*   The reduction in abdominal pressure increases safety for women who have had a previous caesarean section.
*   The support of water enhances the mother's ability to rest more deeply in between contractions. This conserves her energy and strength, giving her greater reserves for a long or difficult labour.
*   There may be less risk of fetal distress.

I am sure that the speakers over the next two days intend to expand on these topics, referring to their research and clinical findings. We can conclude for now that there are more than enough good reasons for women to want to use the birth pool during labour.

I would like now, to introduce some thoughts on the second stage – the birth itself – taking place in water. In the second stage, many women spontaneously stand up out of the water when the baby comes. Often they want to leave the water at the end of labour to give birth on land. They feel they need the security of having their feet on the ground, and the help of gravity when giving birth. It is common that when a mother leaves the pool at the onset of the second stage, no sooner is she standing beside the pool than her baby is born in just a few contractions. However, there are many women who wish to remain in the water to give birth. Generally the percentage of women giving birth in water increases as confidence and experience grows in this way of birthing.

By the end of this conference we will have some idea of the number of babies that have been born in water, both in the United Kingdom and worldwide, and will have had some opportunity to observe the outcomes and safety issues involved.

Since we first heard of the pioneering women who gave birth under water with Igor Tjarkovsky in Russia in the 1960s, and Michel Odent in France in the 1970s, many thousands of mothers all over the world have enjoyed a water birth. My collection of slides includes a mother giving birth in a water pool in a hospital in Japan. Also in Lithuania, where mothers sometimes give birth in the ocean in the summer. Water births have been happening in the Bahamas, Americas and all over Europe. Recently, I took a pool to the northernmost part of Norway where the 'Polar Pool Hire Company' can deliver the pool by helicopter to snow-bound mothers. There are water births happening in Australia, New Zealand, and in fact in every continent on the globe. Here in Britain, by now we can estimate that more than 10,000 women must have laboured or given birth in water.

Thanks to the availability of birth pools, women can now have a water birth in the environment of their choice.

Women, giving birth to their first baby in water, commonly say that at the time they 'knew' intuitively that it was safe and that there was no risk that the baby would drown. While we recognize the need for scientifically based research, let us not discount this motherly intuition as powerful evidence.

This weekend we will learn a lot more about when and how it is safe for a baby to be born in water. We will be hearing from the doctors and midwives who have had the greatest experience of water births both in the United Kingdom and throughout the world. We will learn how the perinatal mortality rate for water births in the United Kingdom compares with the national average for low risk mothers, when speakers from the NPEU present the findings of their recent study.

So, I would like to focus my discussion on the experiential quality of a water birth for mother and baby.

In a water birth, the baby is gently caught and brought slowly to the surface in the first minute after birth.

The first breath is taken once the baby's face comes into contact with the atmosphere. I now know many mothers who have never known another way of birth; who have had two or more water births and cannot imagine giving birth in any other way.

It is usual for these mothers to be ecstatic afterwards. They feel it is the kindest, gentlest and most loving way to have a baby and that nothing could be more natural.

Let us remember for a moment that we all spend the first nine months of our lives in a fluid environment. Very soon after we are conceived, we begin to perceive our bodies through the sensations of warm amniotic fluid on our skin. It is our oldest, most primitive and familiar feeling. Can you imagine what it must be like for a baby to be born in water? If you like, you can close your eyes while you do this.

Imagine being squeezed through the birth canal and then being released by a final reflexive contraction of your mother's womb, through the gateway of her vagina, into the freedom of warm water. Imagine your body suspended, floating, softly held by the water, in what must seem like an infinite ocean of space, and yet gentle and familiar like the warm fluid of the womb. Slowly, your limbs unfold, your body stretching, opening in slow motion, like a flower. For the very first time, your eyes open under the water, and you see a warm, rosy glow of muted light filtering through the pool. Then gentle hands reach down to touch and caress your body softly, inviting, guiding you to the surface, slowly, lifting you up, ever so gently, towards your mother's body. Slowly, your head is brought out into the atmosphere, and there is your mother, your father behind her, gazing at you with eyes of love.

She welcomes you up into her arms, holding you close to her heart against the warmth of her wet, naked body. Cradled safely in her embrace, you begin, in our own time, to gently inhale little breaths of soft, humid air into your lungs, as the rhythmic wave of your breathing begins. Now open your eyes and look at this lovely picture of the first contact between mother and baby in water.

How many of us would like to have been born like this? In my opinion it is easy to understand why women want this sort of birth for their babies.

The continuum, from the womb, through water to the mother's arms, closes the circle. She takes her child right into her heart in the very first moment. The first contact between mother and baby in water has a very special quality. The water enhances the sacred ritual of welcome, the release of emotion, which takes place at this time. When a couple share an experience like this, their baby is born into the protection of a circle of love, which as parents, they will hope to maintain in the years to come.

Sometimes, at a water birth, the whole family is present, including the older children. My own daughters are amongst those fortunate young girls who have had the opportunity to witness such a positive experience of birth during their childhood and adolescence. Let us hope that when they grow up, it will be hard to imagine that we were once afraid to use the simple expedient of the help of water in childbirth.

Water is our friend – it sustains and nurtures all forms of life. It has the power to heal and to bring tremendous benefit to mothers and babies. It is here to help women and midwives as we reclaim the power of birth.

Note: This presentation was illustrated by many slides, including the water labour and births of mothers using the birthing pools produced by the Active Birth Centre, which we were regrettably unable to reproduce in this publication.

CHAPTER THREE

Are We Marine Chimps?

> **Michel Odent** was originally a surgeon. He subsequently became an obstetrician and developed the Maternity Unit in Pithiviers (France), taking into account the importance of environmental factors (first home-like rooms, first birthing pools, and so on). After 1985 he became a midwifery-like practitioner and researcher and founder of the Primal Health Research Centre, and is author of numerous articles and books.

'It is only a passing fad'. This is a comment I often heard in the late 1970s when the media was intrigued by the use of birthing pools in our hospital. In the 1990s the context is different. Hundreds of hospitals, throughout the world, have birthing pools available. When Oxford epidemiologists sent questionnaires to 219 heads of midwifery in England and Wales, it became clear that labour or birth in water – or both – had occurred in all health districts at some time. Today, it is obvious that using birthing pools is not a fad. Those who don't feel comfortable with the attraction labouring women have for water tend to modify their comments, claiming that the use of birthing pools is 'not natural'.

There is reason to pause and reflect on such a point of view, at the very time when a new vision of the origin of *Homo* is developing. Until now it was widely accepted that the crucial factor precipitating the chimpanzee/hominid split was a change in the habitat – from life in trees to life in the great open plains, i.e. the Savannah. This 'Savannah' theory needs to be reconsidered: new dating of the explosion of different species of hoof-footed mammals and pollen analysis led to the conclusion that the great plains and the immense herds on them are relatively recent aspects of the African environment, much more recent than the emergence of *Homo*. This theory also needs to be reconsidered after the recent discovery (1994) by Tim White, of Australopithecus ramidus, still a million years older than the famous Lucy (Australopithecus Afarensis). The fact that the Lucy's bones were found among turtle and crocodile eggs and crab claws has been overlooked. Insofar as it is increasingly difficult to support the Savannah theory, the most basic question regarding human nature must be reformulated: 'Which environment were we - the hominids - originally adapted to?' This issue must be re-explored at a time when molecular biologists claim that we are, so to speak, chimpanzees. We share 98.4 per cent of our genetic material with them. The distance between us and other chimps is less than the distance between gorillas and chimps. According to recent evaluations humans and other chimps separated 'recently', which is no more than 6–8 million years ago. The more the gap between us and chimpanzees is reduced, the more intriguing becomes the morphological and behavioural features that distinguish humans. One way to fathom this mystery is by examining one by one all the features that make humans different from chimpanzees. Such an approach will suggest that there has been probably a time in our evolution when we were adapted to the coast, i.e. to the land-sea interface. This is the basis of the so-called 'aquatic ape theory'.

The most intriguing difference between humans and chimpanzees is brain size: ours is four times bigger than that of our cousin. Nutritionists have an interpretation to offer for this disparity. They have recently realized that there is a family of fatty acids which is essential for the brain. These are the so-called omega 3 polyunsaturated fatty acids. Although they have a precursor in green land vegetables, the polyunsaturated forms are found in the sea food chain only. A large brain – compared with that of genetic relatives – indicates adaptation to the sea. Sea mammals, especially cetaceans, have bigger brains than their cousins on land. This fact provides a new perspective on the primate *Homo*. The human brain combines the structure of the apes' brain with the development of the sea mammals' brain. The nutritional needs of humans in terms of fatty acids suggest that we are primates adapted to the coastal seafood chain. In fact, modern nutritionists claim that humans cannot be totally healthy without occasionally consuming seafood. While, in the past, mothers guided by mere experience knew that cod liver oil was good for their children, there are now scientific reasons for examining the beneficial effects of fish oils in conditions as diverse as heart disease, skin complaints, rheumatism, obesity, diabetes, multiple sclerosis, mental diseases and cancer.

It was this current understanding of our nutritional needs that prompted me to conduct a study of pregnant women who eat a lot of sea fish, especially oily varieties such as mackerel, herring, pilchard, sardines and salmon. We need to know at which point this diet improves the health of pregnant women – and therefore of their babies – influences the way they give birth, and influences the rate of premature births. As the fatty acids of the seafood chain are supposed to facilitate the development of the brain, this long-term project has to follow-up the children.

While our large brain sets us apart from apes, another feature peculiar to humans is the expression of emotion with tears. This is not incompatible with an adaptation to the sea, since marine iguanas, turtles, marine crocodiles, sea snakes, seals and sea otters weep salt tears, while land mammals have no tears or any sort of nasal salt gland. Their existence in humans might be interpreted as a vestige of an extra mechanism for eliminating salt.

The general shape of our body, with the hind limbs forming an extension of the trunk, is not incompatible with aquatic adaptation, since it makes us streamlined, like all sea mammals. The shape of our body is also well adapted for walking and running on two feet. This upright stance is not incompatible with life on the coast: it is easier to keep vertical when moving in shallow water. Human babies, for example, can stay erect and walk in water before being able to walk on dry land.

The absence of hair covering the human body has often been considered as the most striking difference between man and ape. A hairless body is not incompatible with adaptation to the sea. In fact of all mammals we have the highest sweat production. Sweating has long been considered an enigma, or a mistake of nature, as it depletes the body of large amounts of water and salt. This makes no sense at all to those who consider human beings to be first and foremost primates who keep the characteristics of a fetus or a baby until adulthood. (In fact, the human baby does not control its temperature by sweating for the first few weeks following birth.) New interpretations of this sweating mechanism become possible when we consider human beings as primates adapted to environments where water and salt are freely available. In fact, fur seals are the only mammals – apart from humans – who sweat when they are overheated on land: they sweat on their naked hind flippers. Therefore, sweating is another human trait which is not incompatible with adaptation to the sea.

Nose and throat characteristics also offer points of contrast between man and chimp, and even between man and other land mammals. First, we have a prominent nose. Interestingly, the only primate which also has a prominent nose – the proboscis monkey – lives in the coastal wetlands of Borneo and is an excellent distance swimmer. It uses swimming to escape the cloud leopard, which hunts at night and is reluctant to follow its prey into the sea. A long nose is obviously an advantage when swimming or diving, as it deflects water from the nostrils. Another major characteristic of the human face is that we have large empty sinuses on each side of the nasal cavities. The air in these cavities undoubtedly makes our skull lighter, even buoyant, and this too is not incompatible with adaptation to swimming.

Still in the area of the upper respiratory tract, there is another intriguing difference between us and other chimps, and even other land mammals. Our larynx is low, which gives us the choice of breathing with our nose or our mouth. It also allows us to speak. The advantage of a low larynx when swimming is that we can fill our lungs in a second between two strokes. Sea-lions and dugongs are also characterized by a low larynx.

Once again, this is a human feature that is not incompatible with adaptation to the sea. Oddly, however, human beings are not born with a low larynx. Young babies are nose-breathers, which allows them to suck and breathe at the same time. It is around the age of four months that the larynx loses contact with the palate and begins to descend.

While there are many sexual behaviours among land mammals, some general rules do apply. One of these rules is that the male tends to approach the female from behind. In this, humans are special. In most known cultures humans copulate face to face. Moreover, they are orgasmic. Once again, these features are not incompatible with adaptation to the sea, as dolphins and whales also copulate face to face and are very orgasmic. The human vagina shares a number of characteristics with the vagina of sea mammals: both are long and oblique, and both have a hymen. In sea mammals the hymen is supposed to be a barrier preventing water from entering the vagina.

These are only some examples of the features that distinguish humans from other chimps. Of course none of them is sufficient to support the 'aquatic ape theory', but all of them brought together become highly significant. Each feature shows 'no incompatibility' with an adaptation to the sea. That is why this new interpretation of the emergency of *Homo* should be considered as the most serious alternative to the 'Savannah theory'. This vision of homo sapiens was first proposed independently by Max Westenhöfer in Berlin (1942) and by Alister Hardy in Oxford (1960), but it is the British science writer Elaine Morgan who has championed the cause of the 'aquatic ape theory' in her four books. Elaine Morgan also organizes seminars bringing together scientists from a great variety of disciplines, so that the theory is constantly updated, and strengthened. At her last seminar in San Rafael, California, in June 1994, Elaine Morgan proposed an updated comprehensive analysis of the 'Rise and Fall of the Savannah theory'; Derek Ellis, a Canadian professor of marine biology, discussed the possible evolution of pre hominid apes in the formerly flooded Afar triangle; Derek Denton, an Australian professor of physiology discussed interspecies differences in fluid and salt regulation; Michael Crawford, a British professor of nutrition, summarized our current knowledge of the importance of the omega 3 polyunsaturated fatty acids in brain development, while I proposed a new interpretation of pre-eclampsia as the 'primary human disease', and the price we have to pay for having a large brain while we are more or less separated from the sea food chain. The seminar was moderated by Ralph Metzner, who has studied in depth the mythological traces of aquatic human ancestry.

In this new theoretical context, one has great difficulty asserting that the use of birthing pools is not 'natural'. In fact the attraction towards water during labour is not new. It appears that in tropical countries where quiet water was available the place of birth was often close to the river, or the lake, or the sea. The Aborigines of the West Coast of Australia used to walk in shallow water before giving birth on the beach. It is probable that women relaxed and even gave birth in warm calm water in places as far apart as what is today Columbia and Panama, some Polynesian islands, or some Southern Japanese islands. A birth under water was reported in a French medical journal as early as the year 1804. A popular German book, published at the beginning of the century, about 'the mother as a family doctor', indicates how to use a bath during labour.

It is probable that in countries with non-tropical climates the attraction towards water during labour was stifled because hot and cold tap water was not available. However, this attraction could express itself in a subtle way via rituals. Baptism has often been interpreted as a rebirth in water. At the beginning of this century, when most babies were born at home, the father used to spend hours boiling water. This ritual might be seen as an unconscious attempt to include water in birth.

Associating Birth and Water is definitely not new: the goddess of love was born from the foam of the waves!

Further reading

Alderdice, F., Renfrew, M., Marchant, S. et al. (1995). 'Labour and birth in water in England and Wales'. *British Medical Journal*, Vol. 310, p.837.

Crawford, M. (1989). *The Driving Force*. London: Heinemann.

Johnson, J., Odent, M. (1994). *We are All Water Babies*. London: Dragon's World.

Morgan, E. (1932). *The Equatic Ape*. London: Souvenir Press.

Morgan, E. (1990). *The Scars of Evolution*. London: Souvenir Press.

Morgan, E. (1994). *The Descent of the Child*. London: Souvenir Press.

Odent, M. (1983). 'Birth under water'. *The Lancet*, Vol.2, pp.1376-77.

Odent, M. (1990). *Water and Sexuality*. London: Penguin (Arkana).

Odent, M. (1995). 'The primary human disease: an evolutionary perspective', *ReVision*, Washington DC, Vol. 18, No.12, pp.19-21.

PART TWO

The Physiology of Water Birth

CHAPTER FOUR

Water Birth –
A Possible Mode of Delivery?

Gerd Eldering became head of the Obstetric/Gynaecology Department, Vinzenz-Pallotti Hospital in Bensberg Germany in 1980. Since 1982, by vigorously promoting natural and self-determined childbirth under medically safe circumstances in his clinic he became a pioneer of water birth in Germany. He developed his concept in close cooperation with Frederick Leboyer and Michel Odent. The Hospital has 2,000 deliveries a year, and by now more than 2,000 have been water births. Between 1983 and 1987 he conducted a case-control study, comparing the first 1000 water births with 1000 land births of the same parity. Dr Eldering is married and has three children.

Konrad Selke began his medical career with a post-graduate specialization as a paediatrician at the University's Children's Hospital, Medical University of Cologne, Germany. His main working field has been neonatology with emphasis on fetal and neonatal physiology and pathophysiology. Since moving to the Vinzenz-Pallotti Hospital, Bensberg, Germany he has specialized as an obstetrician/gynaecologist. Within the existing team he has been elaborating the main features of water birth physiology, which in fact can be considered to be unique until now. Dr Selke is married and has three children.

Basics

Water birth has been available in Bensberg since 1982. After the first successful (though unplanned) water birth, the number of births underwater has increased over recent years in line with the fluctuations in total deliveries. The percentage of the total births was between seven and twelve per cent, which means between 126 and 216 water births per year, in total numbers. Far from ideological discussions, this contribution aims to give an account of the experiences and discuss theoretical basics (Eldering et al, 1995).

Before introducing the results of our 1000 water births, examined in retrospect, we will briefly explain three areas of fetal and neonatal lung physiology, which are crucial for a water birth (Selke et al, 1995).

Diving reflex

Why does the neonate not normally drown in water? The reason is the diving reflex, an apnoea in expiratory position with closure of the larynx. It is triggered by the receptors of the facial skin and is transmitted by the trigeminus nerve (Tchobroutsky et al, 1969). If this reflex continues to work, a reflex bradycardia commences including a change of the heart minute volume in favour of essential organs.

The diving reflex is different from diving of an adult. During diving the breathing arrest happens in inspiratory position. The diving reflex, however, is similar to the larynx reflexes of the babies, for example when food is regurgitated (Wealthall, 1975; Negus, 1929).

Reflexes submit to a control: in this case a proportional – differential – control. This control reacts to a stimulus with a very rapidly and erratically commencing counter regulation behaviour at first, and then it reaches a different, constant final result, this means that if an adequate stimulus is continuously present during very long phases, there will be an adaptation of the reflex reaction: it leads to intrauterine breathing excursions.

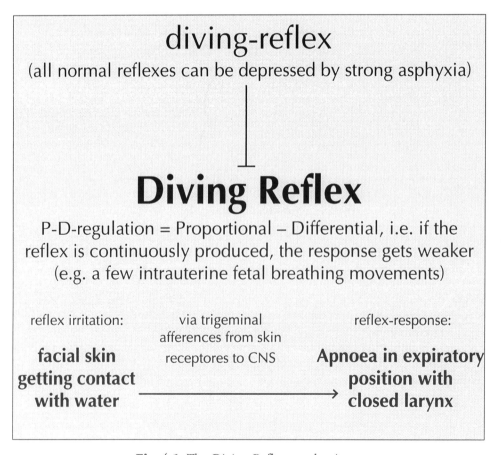

Fig. 4.1: The Diving Reflex mechanisms

Fetal breathing movements

In the beginning it was assumed, of course, that the fetus does not breathe. In 1974 Dawes illustrated by measurement of intratracheal pressures, that lamb fetuses go for regular breathing excursions during the REM sleeping phase (Dawes et al, 1974). Marlet (1970) measured the intraoesophageal pressure as an index for fetal breathing movements. Nowadays there is common agreement that a fetus does practise breathing, starting during early pregnancy. Since there is no exchange of gases, the function is unclear. Dawes (1974) explained that the practice is important for the smooth functioning of the later breathing.

Indeed, we do know that changes of the pattern of the cyclic fetal breathing movement influences the development of the lungs tremendously. Perhaps the movement of the diaphragm and the chest wall cause an expansion stimulus for the lungs and alveolar development?

It has been shown that a bilateral severing of the nervi phrenici (bilateral phrenectomy) leads to decrease of growth of the lungs.

The influence of breathing movements by external stimuli is important. The increased arterial CO_2-partial pressure causes an increase of fetal breathing movements. The intratracheal pressure, the frequency of the movements and the integrated activity of the diaphragm increase. During the high tension electrocorticogram – which represents the NREM-phase – the breathing excursions continue to rest.

Only during unphysiologically high CO_2-tensions (>100mm Hg) and a pH of less than 7.0 was breathing achieved even during the high tension electrocorticogram decreases. We can see a fetal protective and adaptive mechanism. On the other hand, high oxygen tensions of >200mg Hg – applied by 100 per cent oxygen via tube into the fetal trachea – leads to regular fetal breathing movements.

Pharmacological substances, like indomethocine, pilocarpine, 5-hydroxcytryptophan and morphine lead to continuous breathing of different length, independent of the phases of the EEG trace (Hasan et al, 1988) (Figure 4.2).

Fetal lung and fluid

Why does the fetus not aspirate when it makes breathing movements? The answer is simple: the fetal lung is already filled with lung fluid which is produced by itself! The fetal lung epithelium has openings which are smaller than 0.6nm. Thus they form a close barrier against macromolecules. The vascular endothelium, however, has much bigger openings. It therefore allows the passage of bigger protein molecules. The protein contents in the interstitium is, as a result, more than 100 times higher than in the tracheal fluid. Therefore fluid from the lung lumen should flow to the interstitium.

Through an active secretion of chlorid of the lung epithelium there is, however, an osmotic gradient, which allows fluid from the micro circulation to reach the interstitium and then the potential airspace. The lung epithelium actively transports Chloride towards the lung lumen. This process can be stopped by diuretics, which hinder the transport of Chloride which is linked to sodium or potassium.

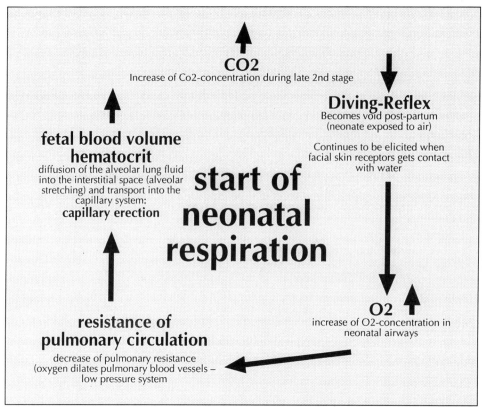

Fig. 4.2: Start of neonatal respiration

In a human fetus about 250–300ml of lung fluid are produced daily. There exists a pressure gradient of 3–5cm H2 above the larynx. During the fetal breathing excursions there is a minimal to and fro movement of the tracheal fluid column. Periodically the larynx opens itself. In this way it allows a net out flow of 15 ml/hr, which is increased about five times during the REM phase.

Ligature of the trachea in utero increases the lung volume. The proliferation and differentiation of alveolar cells increase. Ligature of a branch of the pulmonary artery leads to decreased formation of the fluid on the same side, the lung remains hypo plastic. The same happens with increased drainage of lung fluid, e.g. with oligohydramnios or Pottersequence (the ratio of alveolar cells increases 11:1).

During birth, different hormones increase. The catecholamines especially will be examined more carefully. Thus, the intravenous administration of Adrenaline and Isoproterenol, not of Noradrenaline though, causes the reabsorption of fluid from the lung lumen. This process can be stopped by beta-blockers.

The intraluminal administration of Amiloride – a sodium transport inhibitor – blocks the effect of Adrenaline on the fluid absorption. This observation leads to the assumption that adrenalin stimulates the absorption of sodium by the lung epithelium. This draws, as a result, fluid from the lung lumen to the interstitium.

The fluids get directly absorbed into the bloodstream or it gets drained via the lymphatic system. Zyclo-AMP, injected into the lumen, stimulates the fluid absorption close to the expected date of delivery. Infusions of Arginin-Vasopressin reduce the production of fluid as well as prostaglandin E2. It is likely, therefore, that the reduced fluid production during fetal hypoxia is, at least partially, the result of increased production of stress hormones, which encourages aspiration.

The lung fluid starts to decrease 2–3 days before contractions commence. Therefore the lung fluid of babies born by secondary caesarean section, after the start of contractions, is equally reduced as in babies born vaginally.

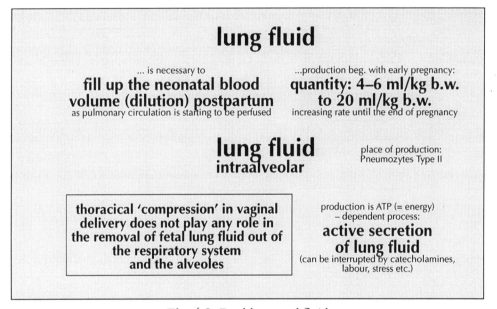

Fig. 4.3: Fetal lung and fluid

Summary

Already in utero the fetus practices breathing. During this time no amniotic fluid gets aspirated into the lungs, but on the contrary a net outflow of lung fluid from the trachea takes place. This mechanism is crucial for the normal growth and differentiation of the lung. The final reabsorption of the fluid is completed within six hours after birth. The vaginal squeezing effect could be ignored (Karlberg et al, 1962).

On the contrary: the newborn needs the lung fluid for his vascular system. He uses it to fill up his intravascular volume, which is increased through opening of the lung system. Postpartum, therefore, the newborn crucially depends on the absorption of lung fluid into his vascular system. When a child is born into water, the diving reflex works completely (Harned et al, 1970). When the umbilical cord pulsates, no reflex bradycardia commences. The lung fluid does not get squeezed out and it does not leave behind a vacuum, but it does get re absorbed as the breathing starts.

With asphyxia, of course, other conditions apply. There is premature fluid absorption and increased breathing activity, which can lead to aspiration.

Material and method

In retrospect, we compared the labour and the neonatal parameter of vitality (Apgar Score) of 1000 water births since 1982, as a control study in 'matched pairs' system.

The control group was formed by subsequent spontaneous births with the same parity.

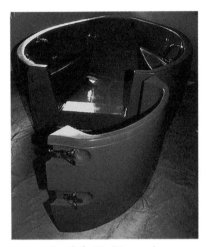

Fig. 4.4: Birthing tub

The aim of this research was to exclude increased risk to mother or baby during an uncomplicated spontaneous birth in water. Only the pregnant woman's wish was decisive as to whether we allowed a water birth - depending on the fetal condition. Further factors, like breech, multiple pregnancy, pathological pregnancies (e.g. placental insufficiency, premature labour before 37/40 weeks gestation) were excluded from delivery in water.

The first 50 births were monitored by continuous CTG - via a scalp electrode. Since then the intermittent control of the fetal heartbeat has been used via an external CTG, as is common for normal spontaneous births (30 minute CTG-monitoring, then one hour without monitoring; if suspect or pathological, shortening of the intervals or continuous CTG). Compare also the relevant statements of American College of Obstetricians and Gynaecologists and Federation of International Gynecologists and Obstetricians for intermittent CTG.

The following parameters were compared between the two groups: age, education, residence, course of pregnancy, history of complications of pregnancy (e.g. previous LSCS), length of contractions, dilatation of the cervix at the beginning of labour, length of stay in the water, use of analgesia during labour, rate of episiotomies/trauma to the birth canal, placental stage, neonatal Apgar scoring and cord-pH, neonatal morbidity (infections, transfers etc.) and mortality, as well as length of hospital stay post partum, were the most important outcomes.

Results: Apgar scoring and cord-pH, neonatal morbidity (infections, transfers etc.) and mortality, as well as length of hospital stay post partum, were the most important ones.

Results

Both groups were homogeneous regarding age, residence, length of the present pregnancy, education, previous pregnancy complications, course of the pregnancy. There was a small increase in the numbers of women in the water birth group who had a history of previous caesarean sections (four per cent to one per cent).

The main part of the delivering women were between 26 and 30 years old. This is in accordance with the statistical age distribution of delivering women in Germany. The majority of women who delivered in water gave birth to their second child.

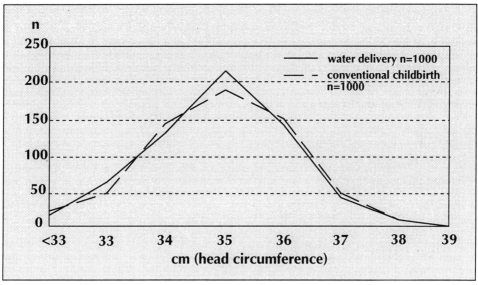

Fig. 4.5: Differences in head circumference between babies born conventionally or in water

The newborn of both groups were not different regarding birthweight and length. The maximum of the distribution graph for the body weight in both groups was around 3500g, the head circumference around 35cm.

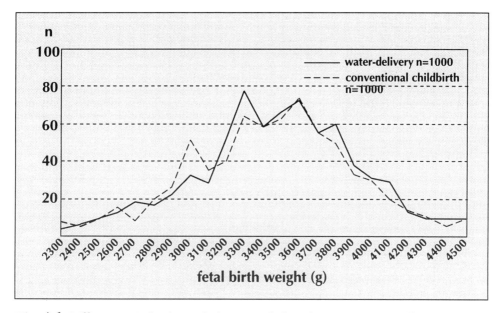

Fig. 4.6: Differences in birthweight between babies born conventionally or in water

Some of the women enter the pool during labour for relaxation, not all of them give birth in water. Only a very small number considered a water birth from the beginning.

Of the women who had delivered in water, 31.5 per cent stayed in the pool for less than one hour, the majority (33.9 per cent) between one and two hours. This means, that two-thirds of the labouring women had delivered after having been in water for two hours.

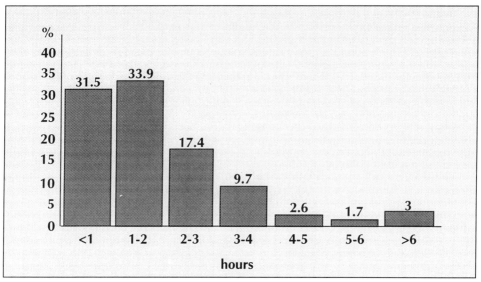

Fig. 4.7: Duration of stay in water

In contrast to other references (Lenstrup et al, 1987) in which the second stage in water is considered to be shorter than during a standard birth, in our comparing groups the length of the expulsion phase was not significantly different. Forty-eight per cent of the water births needed less than 20 minutes, compared with 43 per cent of the control group.

It appeared that relaxation in warm water has a positive result on the pelvic floor. We assume a mental relaxation as well. The vicious circle of tension - anxiety - more tension - increased pain seems to be interrupted more easily in water: we found a significant difference regarding the need for analgesia - 1.1 per cent in water compared with 20.1 per cent outside water.

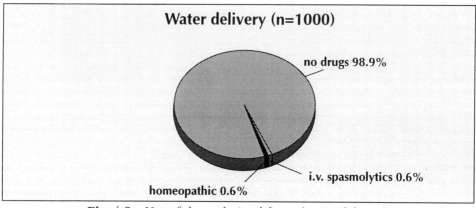

Fig. 4.8a: Use of drugs during labour (water delivery)

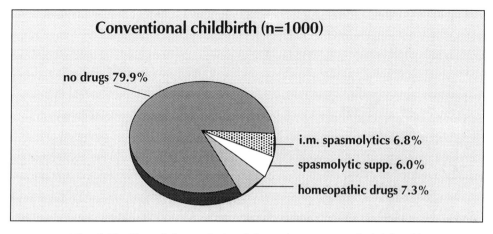

Fig. 4.8b: Use of drugs during labour (conventional childbirth)

If no prophylactic episiotomy is performed, the percentage of episiotomies is around 60 per cent in most obstetric units. We do not cut prophylactically at every birth. The midwife requests an episiotomy only if there is a very tight perineum which might lead to a severe tear or for neonatal reasons.

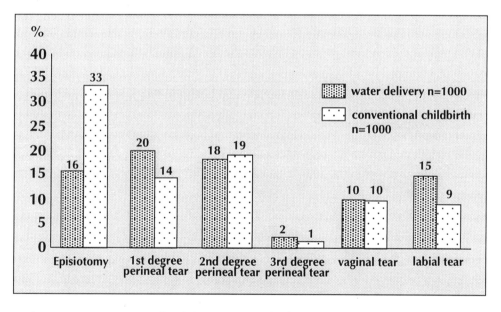

Fig. 4.9: Episiotomy and tear rates

The two groups showed a significant difference regarding the necessary episiotomy, 16 per cent in water and 33 per cent outside water.

A fear of increased haemorrhage during the placental stage caused by dilation of the blood vessels through increased warmth was not proven. Our women determine the comfortable temperature of the water themselves, but we make sure, that the temperature is kept between 32°C and 36°C which is tolerated by the newborn.

The rate of increased haemorrhage was not significant: 12 per cent in water compared with 12 per cent in the control group.

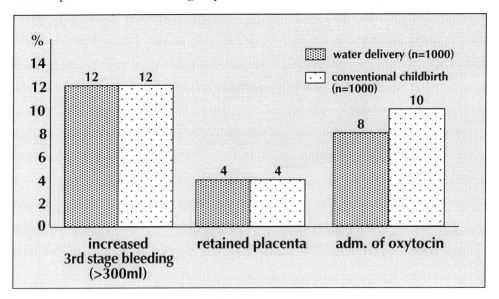

Fig. 4.10: Third stage experiences

The fetal outcome in both groups did not show a significant difference. The distribution of Apgar scores at 1-5 and 10 minutes was nearly identical.

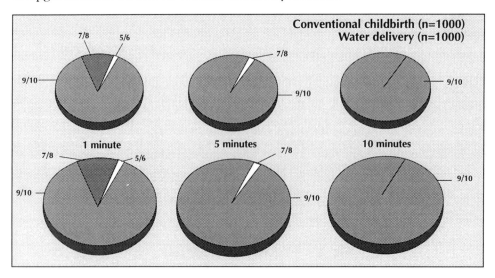

Fig. 4.11: A comparison of apgar scores

Since babies are left undisturbed straight after birth, the conventional ones as well, and since they are not highly stimulated, there were similar conditions.

The arterial cord - pH - values were between 7.2 and 7.29 at 53 per cent of the water births and 46 per cent of the control group. Moderate acidosis occurred in 13 per cent of the water births compared with 14 per cent of the control group.

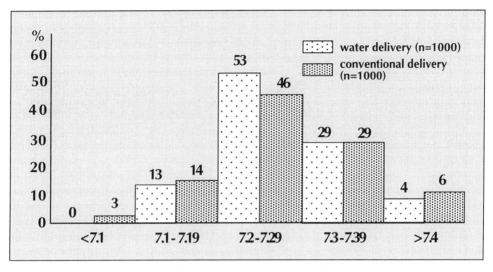

Fig. 4.12: Arterial cord - pH values

Clinical assessment of the newborn did not result in significant differences either. The number of neonatal transfers to the neonatal intensive care unit is low in both groups: 1.1 per cent (water births) and 1.3 per cent (dry land births). There was neither a maternal nor a neonatal death in either group.

There was no profound distribution of volume in the cardiovascular system in our water babies, as Zimmermann (1993) had expected. Our babies were brought to the surface to their mother's breast within five to 40 seconds.

The hospital stay after a water birth was shorter on average, the percentage of domino deliveries was higher.

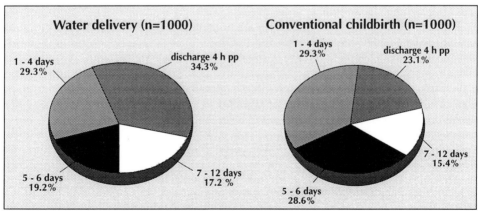

Fig. 4.13: Length of postpartum hospital stay

According to the results of our 1000 water births, examined in retrospect, compared with 1000 spontaneous births outside water, we concluded that no increased neonatal or maternal morbidity or mortality could be shown.

In water the consumption of analgesia was significantly lower (1.2 per cent compared with 20.1 per cent) and the rate of episiotomies less than half. The number of perineal birth trauma, however, was slightly increased in water (53 per cent versus 49 per cent).

Regarding the other parameters examined, there was no significant difference. This is a retrospective study, in which a rather big group was examined regarding this matter. We do not know of a similar research so far, which examines this problem in an equally comprehensive way. A prospective study concerning the same topic is being prepared in our unit.

Criticism of water birth expressed at times is obviously based on assumptions that are not compatible with new insights into fetal physiology and respiratory adaptation of the newborn.

References

Dawes, G.S. et al. (1974). 'Breathing before birth in animal and man'. *New England Journal of Medicine*, Vol.290, p.557.

Eldering, G. et al (1995). 'Entwicklung der alternativen Geburtshilfe am Beispiel der Frauenklinik Bensberg'. In: Siebert, W. Eldering, G. *Alternativen der Klinischen Geaburtshilfe*. Hans Marseille Verlag.

Harned, H. S. Jr., et al (1970). 'The effect of immersion and temperature on respiration in new-born lambs'. *Pediatrics,* Vol.45, p.4.

Hasan, S.U., et al. (1988). 'Effect of morphine on breathing and behaviour in fetal sheep'. *Journal of Applied Physiology,* Vol.64, p.2058.

Karlberg, P. et al. (1962). 'Alteration of the infant's thorax during vaginal delivery'. *Acta Obstetrica Gynecol Scandavia.* Vol.41, p.223.

Lenstrup, C. et al. (1987). 'Warm tub bath during delivery'. *Acta Obstetrica Gynecol Scandavia,* Vol 66, p.709.

Merlet, C. et al. (1970). Mis en evidence de mouvement respiratoirez chez le foetus d'agneau. Cr. *Acad Sci Ser D*, Vol 270, p.2462.

Negus, V.E. (1929) *The Mechanisms of the Larynx*. London: Heinemann.

Selke, K. et al. (1995). 'Wassergeburt-eine mögliche Entbindungsform?' Siebert. W., Eldering, G. *Alternativen der Klinischen Geburtshilfe*. München.

Tchobroutsky, C. et al. (1969). 'The diving reflex in rabbits, sheep and newborn lamb and its afferent pathways'. *Respirat Physiol* Vol.8, p.108.

Wealthall, S.R. (1975). 'Factors resulting in a failure to interrupt apnea'. In Borma, J.F. *Development of Upper Respiratory Anatomy and Function - Symposium.*

Zimmermann, R. et al. (1993). *Die Habamme* Vol.6, p.71.

CHAPTER FIVE

Birth Under Water –
To Breathe or not to Breathe

> **Paul Johnson** is a consultant Clinical Physiologist in the Nuffield Department of Obstetrics and Gynaecology at the John Radcliffe Hospital, Oxford. Most of his research has been on fetal and postnatal neurodevelopment and respiratory control. This has led, in the last five or six years, to the development of portable physiological monitoring systems that can record fetus, mother, and newborn over the telephone lines from wherever they are.

If water births are of psychological and physiological benefit to childbirth, it is logical that this benefit should apply to women at risk during pregnancy too. Therefore what are the risks, if any, of a fetus breathing while under water before surfacing while its umbilical cord is intact? Does it matter that there is a delay before the onset of air breathing? Could the onset of air breathing delayed somewhat by birth under water cause any difficulty to the effectiveness of subsequent breathing?

First of all breathing in fetal life is vigorous, energy consuming, intermittent and obstructed on inspiration. Obstructive apnoea, as it would be called after birth, is essential for lung growth. There is very little inspiration of amniotic fluid. Lung fluid, with very low pH (like gastric fluid) is produced in the lung and is coming out and being swallowed.

Fetal breathing occurs for about 40 per cent of the time in fetal life; its absence, or apnoea, is not to be confused with the diving reflex which can occur as part of a defensive response. The fetus is inhibited from breathing by several mechanisms:

- Hormones, some produced from the placenta and membranes, such as prostaglandin E2, are powerful inhibitors of several brain functions including breathing. About 48 hours before the onset of spontaneous labour fetal breathing stops, while other behaviours and sleep continue. This may be due to the rise in prostaglandin E2 which occurs before labour. Thus an intact placenta and umbilical circulation continues to inhibit breathing even after birth into water.

- The warm temperatures of the fetal environment also acts to inhibit breathing. Environmental heating of the fetus causes panting and cooling stimulates breathing and shivering.

- Metabolism in the fetus is minimal (since the mother provides continuous body warmth). Active thermogenesis or heat production is also inhibited in fetal life (this is unnecessary and potentially harmful because the fetus must lose its heat through the placenta which is relatively slow). Placental hormones probably contribute to this fetal response too. It is important that the mother is not overheated, even if she likes a temperature above her body temperature, since the fetus has no 'choice' in its temperature remaining above that of the mother.

- Hypoxia also inhibits breathing in the fetus, except if very severe, when gasping occurs. Then aspiration of the surrounding liquid could occur.

- People often say that the baby has spent its life immersed in water. This, however, is wrong. It has never experienced water. It has been in amniotic fluid and the fetus knows its ambient conditions better than we do. It senses what is in the fluid. The entrance to the larynx has more taste buds on it than the whole of the tongue. It is bristling with chemoreceptors. This region of the upper airway serves breathing and feeding. It is the key to whether we breathe or swallow. If water replaces amniotic fluid in this region, perhaps by breathing in, breathing is inhibited and swallowing occurs. It would be intriguing if someone described a fetus under water as swallowing rather than breathing. In experiments with lambs they swallowed rather than breathed - and often large volumes if it was water, if it was saline they hardly noticed.

- Water in the larynx causes the diving response - apnoea, swallowing, arousal, bradycardia and hypertension. Blood flow is redistributed to the brain, heart and adrenal glands and this is an important part of this defence response. Many medical drugs, such as atropine and B blockers, stop this happening; they blunt the diving response thus reducing its effectiveness.

- Is it better to be born into sea water or fresh water? The airway chemoreceptors are all round the entrance to the larynx and provide their messages by the superior laryngeal nerve a branch of the vegus nerve. We still do not know what the sensors are, despite the numerous taste buds located precisely in this region. However, there is no apnoea or diving response to saline, amniotic fluid, lung fluid, meconium, gastric fluid, blood, and milk from the same species, and probably sea water (not specifically tested). In other words, the fetus knows its own environmental fluids and body fluids. It equally knows and responds to foreign fluids. Water, foreign milks, alkalis (Coca-Cola, Guinness) cause apnoea. The human infant will swallow and breathe differently when feeding on cows milk or human milk.

In summary, as has been observed in many videos of birth under water, if the onset of labour is spontaneous, and no drugs are administered, a fetus born with its cord intact, into warm, fresh water, not asphyxiated, is inhibited from breathing. Surfacing into cooler, dryer air and clamping of the umbilical cord, then provide the stimulus for it to start breathing.

A full review has been published (Johnson, 1996).

Reference

Johnson, P. (1996). 'Birth under water - to breathe or not to breathe', *British Journal of Obstetrics and Gynaecology,* Vol.103, pp.202-208.

PART THREE

Water Birth and the Family

CHAPTER SIX

Parents' Rights when Choosing to Use a Birth Pool

> **Jayn Ingrey** is the founder of Splashdown Water Birth Services which she formed after a home birth in water of her son, Nathan, in 1989, when she was nearly 35. Jayn has since helped thousands of women to use a water birth pool either at home or in hospital and offers world-wide pool hire. Jayn is one of the organizers of this conference.

I'd like to tell you a little of my involvement with water births which started in 1988, when I first became pregnant with my son Nathan and how this led to the formation of 'Splashdown Water Birth Services', and some of the difficulties women encounter when they want to use a water birth pool, and what their rights are.

I first considered using a water birth pool when I was three months pregnant, and my independent midwife, Jane Davies introduced me to one of her clients who had used a pool. She had been very impressed by the tremendous benefits she had received from labouring in the water and had not needed any additional pain relief. I had been advised of the possible side effects, not just short term, but also long term to both mother and baby, by using pain relief such as epidurals or pethidine. I was, therefore, quite anxious to avoid these, if possible. Due to my age (nearly 35) and the fact that I was unfit and overweight, I felt I wanted to compensate for this by trying to plan the safest and gentlest kind of birth possible for Nathan, and myself, especially as this was my first pregnancy. A water birth at home seemed the natural and obvious choice for me, with options open to transfer to hospital if need be. Also, it meant that Nathan's father could be more involved with the birth. He was responsible for assembling the pool and making sure the water was at the correct temperature. At that time, I didn't realize how uncommon a home birth was, let alone a water birth, because I'd received such fantastic support and encouragement from my midwife. She had previously worked as a community midwife so knew of the advantages of home birth and had also attended several births, where a pool had been used to ease labour. I was also encouraged by reading a full page article in 'The Independent' newspaper in August 1988, during my pregnancy, about Sheila Kitzinger's daughter Tess's home water birth. The photograph of Tess's smiling son Sam, looking into his mother's eyes just after the birth, made a very deep impression on me. Also, the BBC documentary, 'Katy's Birthday', featuring Dr Roger Lichy was shown on television shortly afterwards, showing the last stages of Gill Gribble's pregnancy, her labour in water and Katy's actual birth in the pool. The article and documentary convinced me that I had made the right choice. It also gave me the idea to use the pool not only for pain relief, but actually to give birth in the water as well. Whilst I was in labour, I found it difficult to get into a comfortable position and, although my midwife was very supportive, I found the labour quite agonising. After seven hours, I started to shake uncontrollably in between very strong contractions. That was it - I'd had enough. My options were open, so I decided I wanted to transfer to hospital for an epidural. Fortunately, my midwife persuaded me to get into the pool instead, but at that time, I honestly did not think that a pool of water could help to any great extent as my pains were so intense. I was about six centimetres dilated at the time. However, my midwife promised me that she would take me to hospital if the pool didn't help, and as I was in no frame of mind to argue, I reluctantly agreed. I'm so very glad I did, because on entering the pool the amount of pain relief I received was nothing short of a miracle. I achieved 100 per cent total pain relief instantly. The water was very warm, and my contractions stopped for a minute or two, which gave me time to relax totally and rejuvenate myself. Before the first contraction in the pool occurred, which, thankfully, was about 60 per cent less painful than the previous pains outside the pool, I was able to move freely into any position I liked without discomfort. In the large 5ft circular pool I actually coped with the rest of my labour with comparative ease. I gave birth in the water with Nathan's father sitting next to me in the pool watching the birth into the water. Nathan opened his eyes under the water and seemed to give a little smile. He was lifted gently to the surface and looked straight into my eyes. He was a good pink colour, his Apgar score was 10, and I acknowledged that he wasn't crying, and this seemed perfectly natural to me. He gave a little whimper after a minute or two, and then was perfectly calm again. Little did I know that this experience changed the rest of my life in more ways than one. Not only had I become a mother, but I now had a mission in life!

When I discovered, from Keith Brainen of the 'Active Birth Centre', that I was one of the first women actually to give birth in water in this country, and that there was a need for pool hire and promotion of water birth, I knew I was the woman for the job. I was sure that if such a wonderful birth experience was possible for Nathan and myself, other mothers would also benefit. However, I very naively thought that the promotion of water birth would be an easy task. It seemed so obvious to me that it would be a popular choice when mothers-to-be found out that by relaxing in a luxurious pool of warm water their labour pains would be greatly eased without the potentially harmful side effects of medical pain relief and - yes, many mothers do want to use a pool, but so many are discouraged by their GP, midwife, or obstetrician.

Since forming 'Splashdown' in 1989, I have helped several thousand women to use a water birth pool, despite incredible resistance, just a little of which I will now detail.

The first problem I encountered was that women were told they could not have a water birth in hospital because of the weight of the pools. The weight is not a problem. The water birth pools, weighing anything from a half to one metric tonnes, have been used thousands of times in hospitals, homes, flats and council flats. In fact, I used one of the very heaviest pools in the middle of my first floor room. All 'Splashdowns' pools have been tested by structural engineers for weight distribution. The weight is less than 100lbs per square foot, which is evenly distributed throughout the large pool base area. It can be considered a 'live' load as the pool is only full for a short period of time, as opposed to a 'dead' load such as an x-ray machine or an item that is in one place for a long time. The weight of water birth pools are acceptable for hospitals, houses, and flats, which are designed to take concentrated floor loads of far more than this amount. Another problem women encounter is the difficulty gaining access to the information they need in order to make an informed choice. The 'Cumberlege Report' tells us the woman must be the focus of maternity care. She should be able to feel that she is in control of what is happening to her and be able to make decisions about her care, based on her needs, having discussed matters fully with the professionals involved. There *is* an availability of choice in childbirth, however, women often approach professionals who steer them away from choices they wish to make. I regularly receive calls from women who are told that home birth or water birth is not available to them, especially if they are first time mothers, yet it is these women who are more likely to benefit from home or water birth. Home birth is every woman's right by law. Often women are made to feel intimidated by visits from a midwife and/or Supervisor of Midwives supposedly to fully inform her of the risks. To date, Beverley Lawrence Beech of AIMS informs me that she knows of no instance where the Supervisor of Midwives has fully informed these women of the risks of going into hospital. The women, therefore, have not been fully informed, because the midwives have withheld half the information she would need in order to make a real choice. The following are some examples of the statements women have been given by their midwives:

'The consultant does not advocate water birth',

'But my dear, it's dangerous, don't you know your baby will drown?',

and even 'Who's going to pay for the water?'.

One would assume the same person who would pay for the medical pain relief and anaesthetist's time if an epidural was needed! Midwives can no longer say 'you can't have a water birth because we do not know how to do it,' or 'there is no one here who knows how to do it.' The UKCC' Rules make it clear that the midwife has an obligation to get herself experience and/or education, or seek out someone who is experienced. The Supervisor of Midwives has a duty to ensure that the midwife is adequately prepared and, if she is not, arrange further education and support. Many mothers are concerned that their midwives have agreed to attend their water births reluctantly. This could affect the rapport between midwife and mother and, therefore, the atmosphere at the birth which could affect the labour. Few mothers realize that if they are unhappy with their midwife, at any time during pregnancy or labour, they do have the right to ask to be attended by someone else and the onus is on the Director of Midwifery Services to provide another suitable midwife. However, some mothers feel they have no choice but to pay for an independent midwife. Some mothers try to claim back from the Area Health Authority the fees they were obliged to pay - many unsuccessfully.

In certain hospitals, and indeed home births, where it is perhaps the first, or one of the first, water births in the area, some women have been subjected to curious observers entering the labour room. A woman does not have to be attended by anyone she does not want to be there. Some women who would like to deliver the placenta in the water, find they are told they can't even give birth in the water. Indeed, some women who plan to give birth in the water do decide to leave the pool at the time of birth; and others, who wish to use the pool only for pain relief, may actually give birth in the water, but this should be the woman's choice at the time of birth. However, some Trusts have a policy that the woman should get out of the water for the birth. Many women are intimidated into signing disclaimer forms, as they feel this is the only way they will be able to use a pool at all. This form has no legal status whatsoever and the mother can alter her decision at any time. Any woman who signs a form of agreement who then decides otherwise immediately invalidates her consent. The Trusts have no right to force a woman to leave the pool for the birth and if she refuses, the midwives are obliged to continue with the birth. Pulling out the plug leaves the midwives exposed to a potential legal action for assault. Pumping out the water could electrocute mother and baby, and leaving the room would be seen as neglect. Some Trusts have the idea that they can impose this policy at a home birth. The Trusts have no jurisdiction whatsoever in a woman's own home and their policy is irrelevant.

In January last year, one of my clients, Valerie French, requested a water birth at home for her second baby and was attended by two community midwives. Valerie had used one of my pools before, for the birth of her first child, when it was agreed she could have an underwater birth at home, although, at the time, she decided to leave the pool for the birth. When she became pregnant for the second time, she just said 'I'll have the same again please,' and was even attended by one of the same midwives. This time, however, the midwives were told by their Supervisor that they had to instruct the woman to get out of the water for the birth. This they did, but Valerie said 'Thank you very much, I appreciate your advice, but I think I'd like to stay in the water this time and give birth.' The midwives, confident that they had carried out their Supervisor's instructions, went ahead and delivered the baby. The following day, the Supervisor suspended the midwives and disciplined them. Valerie French reported the story to the media in the hope that justice would be done, but this produced a scare amongst midwives that they could be suspended if they attended a water birth. The lead midwife who attended Valerie French's birth is now working for another Area Health Authority, and the Supervisor of Midwives is now herself the subject of a complaint to the UKCC.

One woman phoned me recently, delighted with her baby and said that the pool had been wonderful. When I asked if she had given birth in the pool she said she would have done, but just as she was about to give birth the Supervisor of Midwives entered the room and pointed at one of the attending midwives bellowing 'Get that woman out of that pool now.' Unfortunately, the woman did reluctantly agree. She need not have done so.

I would like to see a future where professionals provide complete, up-to-date and unbiased information on the choices available to women. It's their bodies, their babies, and they have the right to choose where and how they give birth, but in order to do this they must have information.

Information is power, the power enables women to make choices for themselves.

CHAPTER SEVEN

Water Births in a Rural Community

Roger Lichy is an independent General Practitioner using Classical Homeopathy to treat mainly chronic diseases. He has a special interest in obstetric homeopathy and teaches this in London and Prague. He enjoys attending childbirth at home and introduced water births to Cornwall in 1985. He wrote *The Waterbirth Handbook* and helped to popularize water births by appearing in the press, radio and television. He is currently taking a Master's Degree in medical anthropology.

I have decided to take some liberties with the title of this talk and rather than analyse my water birth data, the conclusions of which are much the same as those we have already heard today, I would like to talk about just one of my water births. This is the case history of Maria, a mother who had a five hour progressive slowing of first stage labour, and a three hour arrest at eight to nine centimetres cervical dilatation. Administration of the correct homeopathic remedy stimulated normal labour and she proceeded to have a normal water birth at home, thereby avoiding a transfer to the hospital obstetric unit, a journey which can take over an hour in the busy summer months.

First though, I would like to describe my practice and its location. For the past twenty years, I have been a General Practitioner (GP) in Penzance, a small town at the extreme south-west tip of England, some ten miles from Land's End. I was part of the National Health Service (NHS) in the early years of practice and made good use of our local sixteen bed GP maternity unit. By 1982, however, I had become increasingly dissatisfied with the biomedical treatment of disease and left the NHS, retrained in homeopathy and became an independent GP. Leaving the NHS gave me the opportunity to start a domiciliary childbirth service in West Cornwall, a birthing option all the more appreciated by local women with the closure of the local GP maternity unit in 1987 and the nearest obstetric unit at Treliske Hospital some twenty five miles away. The relative geographic isolation, coupled with an enthusiastic community midwifery service, has resulted in the Penzance area having a high domiciliary birth rate - approximately 25 per cent in 1993.

In 1985, I attended my first water birth after which the mother gave me her purpose-built pool, saying that she wanted me to have it so that other women could experience the same benefit that she had found while labouring in warm water (Lichy and Herzberg, 1993). Now nearly 100 childbirths later, the pool is still in use, though relegated to backing up a more recently acquired pool.

I regard myself as primarily a homeopathic GP who specializes in obstetrics and obstetric homeopathy. More than 95 per cent of the medicines that I use in my practice are homeopathic remedies which I find to be more effective, safer, and less expensive than conventional medicines. Homeopathic treatment is started as early as possible in pregnancy so that the mother is in the best possible state of health for childbirth. Taking her homeopathic case history also gives me some idea of what homeopathic remedies might be needed in labour itself, although my aim is for the mother to deliver without any interventions from me. I find homeopathy to be particularly effective in treating complications in pregnancy such as nausea, hypertension and oedema, complications of labour such as maternal distress and failure to progress, and complications in the postnatal period such as depression and mastitis.

Let us get back to Maria. I first saw her in November 1992, eight weeks pregnant. She was a thirty-two-year-old devout Roman Catholic woman, of Italian immigrant parents, and had two children, Francesca aged four and Marco aged two. Maria's first child was induced at 41 weeks for post-maturity by means of an artificial rupture of membranes (ARM) and Syntocinon drip with a resulting vaginal delivery of an undiagnosed breech baby, birth weight 3400g. Her second child, who also had a birth weight of 3400g, was induced at 42 weeks, again for post-maturity, again with an ARM and Syntocinon. This time though, she ended up with a caesarean section because at low levels of Syntocinon infusion she had no contractions and with levels sufficiently high to produce contractions, there was fetal distress. She was told there was placental insufficiency. An interesting feature of both births is that Maria did not have a single contraction without the aid of syntocinon, not even any Braxton-Hicks contractions, in either of her pregnancies.

Maria wanted to have her third child at home. She adamantly refused even to consider having another hospital birth, saying that during her last childbirth she 'was never so frightened in my life with all the doctors squabbling in the room, I panicked ... (and) said my Hail Mary's out loud.' She spontaneously added, 'I hated all the doctors and midwives coming in every half hour doing examinations, every one of them different, I hated it when they just barged in'. I agreed to attend her home birth only on the condition that I could find a homeopathic remedy which would enable her to start off in normal labour at term without the need for an ARM and Syntocinon.

She had an uneventful pregnancy, apart from some early nausea which was relieved by a single oral dose of the homeopathic remedy Phosphorus 200. At thirty four weeks, she began to experience Braxton-Hicks contractions which she had not done in her previous pregnancies. By forty weeks, she was having uncomfortable half hourly contractions and was given a single dose of Phosphorus 10M to try and initiate labour in view of the past history of placental insufficiency. This was unsuccessful and two days later she was started on Caulophyllum 30, one every twelve hours. She reported that 'very soon' after taking the first Caulophyllum tablet, she noticed an increase in frequency of her contractions and forty eight hours later she was woken from sleep at 23.00hrs. with painful contractions every ten minutes.

Caulophyllum is a homeopathic remedy prepared from the Blue Cohosh, a North American plant known as 'Squaw Root' by native Americans because of its herbal reputation for easing difficult births. I chose this remedy for Maria because it is known to be effective for mothers with mild anticipatory anxiety about the outcome of pregnancy (Moskowitz, 1992). At 36 weeks, although Maria did not display any overt signs of anxiety and stated that she was feeling confident, she did admit to 'momentary worries' about the future birth and that 'if it were to go wrong, I'd panic'. Caulophyllum is the most commonly used of about a dozen or so different homeopathic remedies which are known to initiate labour, only one of which will be effective for a particular mother at a particular time. Had Maria been in an extremely anxious, irritable, morose state of mind, I would have chosen a different remedy for her, perhaps Cimicifuga prepared from Black Cohosh. The selection of the correct remedy depends on the psychological and the physical state of the mother; the administration of the correct remedy relieves the dysphoria producing the abnormal physical state.

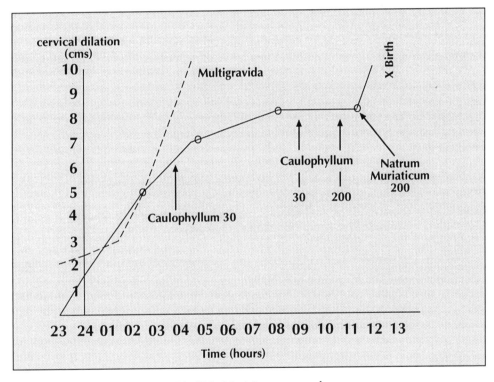

Fig.7.1: Maria's partograph

As you can see from her partograph (Fig.7.1), Maria started off well and her cervix dilated faster than average. At her first examination at 02.20hrs, soon after I arrived at her house, her cervix had opened up some five centimetres in just over two hours. After this promising start, the curve gradually flattens out as the cervix opened up more and more slowly, until it became fixed at eight to nine centimetres for some three hours. From the time of my arrival, her contractions were moderately strong and irregular, occurring every three to seven minutes. After the birth, when asked how she felt during this time, Maria said that her contractions were, 'getting less painful as time went on, I thought that everything was slackening off, that it was stopping'. Abdominal palpation was normal, the fetal heart rate was steady at around 140 and the membranes were intact.

I first of all tried repeating Caulophyllum on the basis that as it had worked well in stimulating her uterus to begin with, it was worth spending some time making sure that the remedy had not just 'worn off', with a return of her concern about the outcome of her labour. Eventually, I was forced to the conclusion that Caulophyllum was not the correct remedy for her during this phase of labour, especially after repeating it in a higher dose.

After careful observation of Maria, I gave her a single dose of Natrum Muriaticum 200 at 11.15hrs. This was immediately followed by five consecutive strong contractions at three minute intervals (the first three minute contractions of her labour), causing her to comment, 'this is the worst [pain] yet - it's horrible'. At 11.41hrs, she was becoming distressed by the pain and went into the water tub. At 11.50hrs she wanted to push and examination confirmed that she was fully dilated. She had a second stage of 27 minutes and delivered a 3550g male who cried immediately and had an Apgar of ten at one minute. The placenta was normal with no sign of insufficiency. Blood loss was 200ml. She had a small ventral tear repaired with one suture.

In summary, she had progressive slowing and arrest of labour for almost nine hours. She had a single dose of Natrum Muriaticum with a normal birth of her child in water one hour later.

Why did her labour slow down and stop? On the physical level, everything appeared to be normal, but what about Maria's psychological state? Could she have been experiencing some inner turmoil which was inhibiting her cervical dilatation? At first sight, this seems unlikely. During the whole of her observed labour up to the time of giving her the Natrum Muriaticum, she appeared to be in a peaceful and relaxed state both during and between her contractions. For the majority of the time, she sat quietly and composedly in an armchair close to mine, occasionally getting up to walk around the room or to go to the bathroom. She spoke very little, mainly in reply to one of the three other people in the room (her husband, her sister and myself) but when she did speak, her voice and content were unremarkable. She made no spontaneous comments about herself or her labour during this period and she remained totally silent during her contractions. Neither her posture nor the expression on her face changed in the slightest, the only indication that she was experiencing a contraction was that she closed her eyes.

If asked to describe Maria's behaviour, the most appropriate word would be 'private'. With hindsight, this theme of privacy can be seen to run through her life. First, her complaints about the lack of privacy in hospital, 'all the doctors and midwives coming in every half hour... they just barged in', was one of the main reasons for her choosing a home birth. Each time that I checked her cervix, she requested her husband and sister to leave the room in order to be as private as possible during the examination. Even the spatial arrangement of her husband and sister in the birthing room indicated this need: she sat in one corner of the room and by some sort of unspoken language her husband and sister spent the majority of the time sat on a sofa ten feet away from her. She did not want any physical contact with them or me. She sat enfolded by the barrier-like back and sides of the armchair, as if it were a protection against anyone coming too close to her.

It was the observation of her stoic behaviour and the realization that here was a woman with intense privacy of her thoughts, emotions and body language led me to select Natrum Muriaticum for Maria. This need for privacy is one of the hallmarks of the Natrum Muriaticum personality, for it is only in privacy and solitude that they can be free of the anxiety of worrying what others are thinking of them (Coulter, 1988). Privacy is demonstrated on all levels of life: on the emotional level, they prefer to cry alone, on the mental level they prefer to be alone to work or create, and on the physical level they like to take long solitary walks, preferably in the country.

Given that she was an extremely private person and a devout Catholic, what hidden emotion could she have been experiencing to such an extent that it was inhibiting her cervix from opening? I did not know at the time and it was only on reflection after the birth that I realized that it must have been embarrassment: her embarrassment at having to display her genitalia during vaginal examination to a comparative stranger, embarrassment at being digitally penetrated whilst her cervix was assessed, embarrassment at the thought of her genitalia being the forthcoming object of gaze when her baby emerged. When directly asked after the birth, Maria confirmed this notion by saying, 'The examinations, I hated all that, it's the worse thing about it all, I get really, really, embarrassed at anyone doing an examination. That's the reason I always refuse smear tests and why I always take my own stitches out before the midwife comes on the sixth day, so she won't have to do it'. To all of us brought up in the Judeo-Christian-Islamic tradition, our body and bodily functions are a cause of embarrassment to a greater or lesser extent, but what I am suggesting here is that in Maria's case these feelings were so overwhelming that they prevented her from 'letting go' and relaxing her cervix. After taking Natrum Muriaticum, her embarrassment subsided to manageable levels and her cervix relaxed.

Vithoulkas (1986) describes something similar in the male Natrum Muriaticum personality in that he may have difficulty urinating when he thinks that he is being watched. For example, he may go to the cinema and drink a large coke while watching the film. At the end of the programme, he has a full bladder and joins the queue in the men's toilet waiting for an empty urinal. When his turn comes, he stands at the urinal, waiting for his bladder sphincter to relax so that he can pee. Now the Natrum Muriaticum personality is so sensitive to what others might be thinking about him that he imagines the man waiting in the queue behind him is thinking, 'I wish that chap would hurry up and start peeing so that I can have my turn'. And the embarrassment at the thought of being watched and criticized while trying to urinate makes it impossible for him to relax his bladder sphincter and start urinating. The more he tries to contract his bladder to force out his urine, the harder his sphincter contracts. Eventually he gives up and slips into an empty toilet cubicle, if available, locks the door and has no difficulty at all in urinating in privacy.

To women who are in this pattern the thought of another person seeing their genitals, even in the supposedly non-sexual context of childbirth, can be as embarrassing as being asked to masturbate openly in public. Of course, there are both men and women to whom this might be an exciting challenge but we are not talking about people who crave sexual stimulation. The typical Natrum muriaticum person is sensitive, self-conscious, self-critical, perfectionist and reserved (Vermeulen, 1992).

Finally, there is the disturbing thought that, even if I had not examined her at all, would labour have stopped just by my sitting in a chair next to her, in much the same way that Natrum Muriaticum males find it impossible to relax and urinate in the close physical proximity of others? As Sheila Kitzinger said in a newspaper article a few weeks ago, 'Some women need to be solitary ....during labour' (Kitzinger, 1995).

References

Coulter, C.R. (1988). *Portraits of Homeopathic Medicine*. Berkeley, California: North Atlantic Books.

Kitzinger, S. (1995). *The Observer*, March 12, London.

Lichy, R., Herzberg, E. (1993). *The Waterbirth Handbook*, Bath, UK: Gateway.

Moskowitz, R. (1992). *Homeopathic Medicines for Pregnancy and Childbirth*. Berkeley, California: North Atlantic Books.

Vithoulkas, G. (1986). *Homeopathy for the New Man*. Bath, UK: Thorsons.

PART FOUR

Technology and Childbirth

CHAPTER EIGHT

Is Obstetrics Good for Your Health?

Beverley Lawrence Beech is a freelance writer, campaigner, mother of two and Chair of the Association for Improvements in the Maternity Services. She regularly lectures internationally to lay audiences and midwifery schools, and often appears on radio and television. For six years she was a lay adviser to the National Perinatal Epidemiology Unit at Oxford. In November 1994 she was appointed to the Midwifery Committee of the United Kingdom Central Council for Nurses, Midwives and Health Visitors. She is the author of *Who's Having Your Baby?* and co-author, with Jean Robinson, of *Ultrasound? Unsound.* Beverley is one of the organizers of this conference.

'The ability to intervene effectively to determine the timing of a human birth gives the obstetrician a heady feeling of power, he should therefore approach the use of this clinical weapon (induction of labour) with extra circumspection and always be conscious of the temptation to interfere for inappropriate reasons.' (Calder, 1991).

Judging by the numbers of women who book into large, centralized obstetric units every year, the answer to the question 'Is obstetrics good for your health?' is yes. Examine the literature and consider the reasons for the majority of obstetric interventions, the answer has to be no.

If you read Marjorie Tew's book *Safer Childbirth?* you will see that her analysis of childbirth statistics revealed that had women stayed at home to have their babies the infant mortality rates would be four points lower than they are now. That means that every year 2,400 babies in the United Kingdom could be dying as a direct result of their mothers choosing to give birth in hospital.

Technologies developed to help babies and mothers with problems were very quickly transferred and used on the majority. Active Management of Labour, a means of accelerating labour, a pattern which was based on the duration of labour based on the obstetricians' limits, not on the woman's or the baby's was soon used on almost everyone. In Dublin where over 6,000 babies are born in Holles Street Hospital alone, it was a very useful tool by which the women could be processed through the baby factory as quickly as possible. As the numbers of births went up so the length of time the women were allowed to labour went down.

The doctors developed industrial line management techniques and applied them to labouring women. In order to get the women to accept this level of interference they persuaded them that they would guarantee that no labour lasted longer than 12 hours, and to ensure that they gave every woman the constant company of an obstetric nurse. The vast majority of the antenatal classes are run by the hospital's midwives, so they ensure that the women are programmed to accept what is on offer, and they have very few uppity women questioning the status quo.

At a meeting of obstetricians and lawyers in the USA the moderator reminded the audience that *'Oxytocin has done more to raise the living standards of medical malpractice attorneys than any other drug on the market.'* (Haire, 1994).

Throughout pregnancy women are exhorted not to drink alcohol, smoke or take drugs, because of anxieties about the potential effects on the baby. Yet the moment a woman steps inside a labour ward she is subjected to a battery of interventions and drugs, most of which have not been studied for their long term effects, and by long term we mean 10, 20 and 30 years.

There have been enough disasters to alert us to potential hazards yet we persist in playing down the possible and even known risks.

In the 1960s, 4,650 babies were born suffering from the side effects of Thalidomide, a drug given to women during their pregnancies. In 1993 a baby was born in England to a Thalidomide father, she was his third child and the other two were completely normal. This baby has exactly the same abnormalities of her hands and feet as her father. Two generations affected by the same drug.

In America, the grandchildren of women who took Diethylstilbestrol during their pregnancies, in the misguided belief that it would prevent miscarriage, are now suing the pharmaceutical company for the damage they are suffering as a result of the abnormalities of the genital tract their mothers' suffered. This is a third generation.

By failing to take heed of these warnings we could be laying up problems for future generations. What are the long-term effects of oxytocin, syntometrine, morphine or epidural bupivicaine, to name but a few of the very powerful drugs that are routinely used in an obstetric unit? Modern obstetric care is far too cavalier in its attitude to intervention, and it is time we took action. We will never wrest the toys from the boys, but we can ensure that they are used as little as possible.

We had hoped that proper evaluation of medical technology and drugs would result in changes in practice. Unfortunately, knowledge of the research appears to have little effect when it reveals that the toys are not as wonderful as the boys thought. Electronic fetal monitoring is a classic example. It was developed to enable doctors to tell what was happening in the womb without having to rely on the woman. To achieve this most women are confined to a bed, flat on their backs, or in a semi-recumbent position. What is disturbing about electronic fetal monitoring is the blind trust the midwifery and medical staff have in its efficacy. Despite nine randomized controlled trials demonstrating that it does not work, cannot be certain to be interpreted with any accuracy, and on the occasions where it does work correctly the hospital staff can fail to respond.

There are thousands of midwives and doctors throughout the UK who have convinced themselves that they can interpret the print outs. Yet when a study was conducted of acknowledged experts from a number of different countries who were sent the same selection of print outs they returned a wide variety of interpretations, and when they were sent the same printouts six months later they gave different interpretations. A further study (Keegan, Waffarn and Quilligan, 1985) showed 37 per cent of tracings to be difficult or impossible to interpret.

And what effect does electronic fetal monitoring have on the baby? The nine randomized controlled trials have shown no differences in Apgar score at birth, cord blood gases at birth, the need for newborn intensive care and long-term neurological status. A randomized clinical trial of premature babies, of which one group had EFM and the other did not, revealed that the monitoring group suffered a 20 per cent cerebral palsy rate while the auscultation group suffered an 8 per cent cerebral palsy rate (Shy et al, 1990).

The Dublin trial showed fewer seizures in the monitoring group, but further analysis revealed that the seizures occurred mainly in women who had had oxytocin to induce or accelerate their labours, and when oxytocin cases were removed there was no difference in the seizure rates in both groups. Furthermore, a follow-up study a year later showed no difference in the numbers of neurological handicaps in each group (MacDonald et al, 1985).

Doctors persist in using electronic fetal monitoring, not only because the toys appeal to the boys, but also because they believe it protects them from litigation, apparently unaware that fetal monitoring traces have given the parents considerable ammunition over the years.

We do not know how many babies have contracted HIV and developed AIDS as a result of the use of electronic fetal scalp electrodes, but it was some time after AIMS first warned of the risk that the medical profession began to discuss that connection. Their response has been interesting, they are now developing a non-penetrating scalp electrode. Only now is the profession talking about the risk of scalp abscesses (0.3-5.4 per cent), sepsis, cerebro-spinal fluid leakage and the risks of transmitting HIV and other infections (Hofmeyr et al, 1993). Few mothers are told that in order to attach a fetal scalp electrode a double ended needle has to be screwed into the baby's scalp.

While electronic fetal monitoring persists midwives are being de-skilled, and there are some midwifery schools which now actively discourage the midwife from developing her skills in listening to the fetal heart rate with a Pinard stethoscope. Much better to encourage her to use a sonicaid and expose the baby to yet more Doppler ultrasound. AIMS became concerned about the possibility of harmful effects of ultrasound in the late 1970s, when we obtained research papers from the USA suggesting that ultrasound was not absolutely safe. In 1982 Liebeskind et al published a paper in the British

Journal of Cancer of the cellular effects of pulsed diagnostic ultrasound and concluded, *'The persistence of abnormal behaviour and motility in cells exposed to a single dose of diagnostic level ultrasound ten generations after insonation suggests permanent hereditary effects. .. It is not known whether the in vitro effects of ultrasound also occur in vivo.'* Apart from one or two clinicians (Bases, 1990) the medical profession has dismissed Liebeskind's findings on the grounds that they could not be repeated by other researchers and claim that *'it is generally accepted that when used by competent qualified personnel, current diagnostic imaging equipment operating in a scanning mode will not cause significant biological effects in mammalian tissue'* (De Crespigny, 1990).

When we talk about *'diagnostic levels of ultrasound'* we should make it clear that these are usually not measured, and they vary widely between different machines and different makes. Users do not actually know the extent of exposure a baby is receiving from any individual machine.

Trans-vaginal ultrasound is now being developed. A probe is inserted into the vagina so that the ultrasound can be nearer to the baby. This is being widely used for research, monitoring development of the fetal brain and organs from the earliest stages. We see many published research papers where studies have been done on movements of the fetus in utero, e.g. breathing, thumb sucking, swallowing etc. which are carried out for up to an hour or more at a time. No concern is expressed about possible damage or the need for long-term assessment of exposed infants, or what possible value there is in this superficial kind of research.

Babies in special and intensive care baby units are frequently (often many times a day) exposed to lengthy examination of their brains by ultrasound. What are the long-term effects on these babies?

In a Finnish study, recently published in The Lancet (Saari-Kemppainen, 1990), of 30 apparently abnormal babies detected by ultrasound, 10 later proved to be normal. AIMS knows of a number of cases where ultrasound diagnosis of congenital abnormality has resulted in the abortion of a fetus which proved to be perfectly normal. Mothers are not always told this has happened, and they carry into subsequent pregnancies their anxiety about the previously 'abnormal' baby. In a recent case, a woman telephoned us to say that she had had a scan and the doctor told her that the baby was a dwarf and they would arrange for an abortion. She did not believe them and refused. She was short and so was her husband, so she saw no reason why her baby should not be short also. She subsequently gave birth to a perfectly normal baby.

We are told that screening is reassuring for women. Of 250 women diagnosed by ultrasound as having placenta praevia in the Finnish study, only four had the condition at delivery. The unnecessary anxiety caused to the remaining 246 women can hardly have been negligible and, unfortunately, is rarely investigated.

We have cases of women who are sure of the date of conception, but are told that ultrasound tests have proved them wrong. The baby is induced because obstetricians say the pregnancy has gone way beyond term, but a premature baby is in fact delivered and in some cases died. Conversely, we have cases where the woman is saying she is overdue and is not believed, because the ultrasound was believed to show a different expected date of delivery. In one such case, a woman was given drugs to suppress what the staff believed to be a premature labour, despite her protests, and a full term fetus was tragically delivered dead.

'Studies of the efficacy of ultrasonography in pregnancy have not been encouraging. Such screening has not been shown to have any benefit either as a single or as a two stage procedure, apart from reducing the number of women induced for incorrectly diagnosed post-maturity' (Cahill, 1991).

There is *'no statistically significant reduction in perinatal morbidity and mortality associated with the routine use of ultrasound'* (Thacker, 1985).

It is presumed that it is better to abort a seriously damaged baby rather than support the parents through the birth, but no comparative studies have been done. Parents who gave birth to live babies with fatal abnormalities who took them home and cared for them until they died weeks or months later felt that they had benefited from an opportunity to know and grieve for a child whom they had known. Of course perinatal or infant mortality statistics are less satisfactory if the child is not aborted, but recovery from grief in the family may in some cases be better if the child is born and dies later. The emotional impact on the family which has taken the decision to abort a baby with fetal abnormalities has been little studied but we can report the comment of one mother who said 'What I have to live with is the knowledge that I killed my baby.'

Adequate research has not been done on the long term consequences of decisions to abort or not to abort.

A randomized controlled trial by Newnham et al (1991) using Doppler ultrasound revealed that the exposed babies were more likely to suffer fetal distress after induction of labour leading to emergency caesarean section and were more likely to have depressed Apgar scores at birth.

In 1992 Davies et al published the results of a randomized controlled trial of Doppler ultrasound in Queen Charlotte's Hospital four times as many babies died in the Doppler group. It is interesting to note that while the medical profession was vigorously demanding a stop to water births following the death of one baby they remain totally silent about the sixteen deaths in this study. Clearly, it is not the pile of dead bodies that provokes them into action.

No one is suggesting we lock up the drugs and the technology and let the women get on with it. There are women and babies who need these medical interventions. The tragedy is that the medical profession's take-over of normal birth has resulted in all women being subjected to these methods. So successfully have women been brainwashed into accepting obstetric interventions they feel they have been deprived if they have not had them. Anyone who has read our national papers over the last few weeks will have seen articles and letters from women who have had dreadful experiences giving birth and have convinced themselves that they have had a normal birth. What they had was an vaginal delivery which followed the standard obstetric interventions.

In 1760 a midwife, Elizabeth Nihell, wrote: *'he (the doctor) used instruments unnecessarily to hasten the birth and save his own time, as well as to impress the family with his dexterity and justify charging a higher fee. .... Worse still, the male practitioner, adding insult to injury, was so adept at concealing his errors with "a cloud of hard words and scientific jargon" that the injured patient herself was convinced that she could not thank him enough for the mischief he had done'* (Donnison, 1977).

What has changed?

It is time midwives stopped the practice of writing *'normal delivery'* on the case notes of a woman who has had artificial rupture of membranes, an oxytocic drip, pethidine, epidural anaesthesia and an episiotomy.

What they should write is vaginal delivery - technological labour. Then perhaps midwives and mothers will begin to understand the differences between a normal birth and a technological birth. Unfortunately, it is not the mothers who need educating, there are many midwives who haven't seen a normal birth in years and are as unaware as the mothers.

For the majority of women we have to develop alternatives to drugged and technological births. We cannot simply withdraw the drugs and let the women get on with it, when they are going into a high technology unit where the staff have no conception of normal birth. We have to offer an alternative form of care which is supportive, nurturing and sensitive to the women's needs.

Water birth is an alternative to drugs, and, so far, it has no known side effects, and it has the added advantage of making the woman more difficult to get at. As with all new techniques we want water birth to be properly evaluated. Had obstetricians been as eager to publicize the side effects of drugs, and other treatments, as they have been to draw attention to the problems they perceived with water birth very few of their current practices would have got off the ground.

We will never get all women out of hospital, but we can work to minimize the negative effects an institution has, but don't make the mistake of believing that this will be 'just like a home birth', it won't, but it can come close.

References

Bases, R. (1990). 'Should all pregnant women be offered an ultrasound examination?' *The Medical Journal of Australia,* Vol.152, 21 May 1990, p.557.

Cahill, D.J. (1991). 'Ultrasound and perinatal mortality rates' *British Medical Journal,* March 16, Vol 302, p.662.

Calder, A. A. (1991). 'Reasons for and methods of induction of labour. *Journal of Obstetrics & Gynaecology,* Vol.11, (Suppl 1), S2-S5.

Davies, J. et al. (1992). 'Randomised controlled trial of doppler ultrasound screening of placental perfusion during pregnancy'. *The Lancet,* Vol.2, pp.1299-1303.

De Crespigny, LCh.(1990). 'Should all pregnant women be offered an ultrasound examination?' *British Medical Journal,* Vol.302, p.662.

Haire, D. (1994). 'Obstetric Drugs and procedures: their effects on mother and baby' *AIMS Australia Quarterly Journal* Vol.1, No.6.

Hofmeyr, G.J., Nikodem, C., Gülmezoglu, A.M., Bunn, A.E. (1993). 'A nonpenetrating fetal scalp electrode', *British Journal of Obstetrics and Gynaecology,* Vol.100, pp.649-652.

Keegan, K., Waffarn, F., Quilligan, E.J. (1985). 'Obstetric characteristics and fetal heart rate patterns of infants who convulse during the newborn period', *American Journal of Obstetrics and Gynaecology,* Vol.153, pp.732-737.

MacDonald, D., Grant, A., Sheridan-Pereira, M., Boylan, P and Chalmers, I. (1985). 'The Dublin randomized trial of intrapartum fetal monitoring', *American Journal of Obstetrics and Gynecology,* Vol.152, pp.524-539.

Newnham, J.P. et al. (1991). 'Doppler flow velocity waveform analysis in high risk pregnancies: a randomized controlled trial', *British Journal of Obstetrics and Gynaecology,* Vol.98, pp.956-963.

Nihell E. (1977). Quoted by Donnison, J. in *Midwives and Medical Men. A History of the Struggle for the Control of Childbirth.* p.44.

Shy, K., Luthy, D.A., Bennett, F.C., Whitfield, M., Larson, E.B., van-Belle, G., Hughes, J.P., Wilson, J.A,. Stenchever, M.A. (1990). 'Effects of electronic fetal-heart-rate monitoring as compared with periodic auscultation, on the neurological development of premature infants', *New England Journal of Medicine,* Vol.322, No.9, pp.588-594.

Saari-Kemppainen A et al. (1990). 'Ultrasound screening and perinatal mortality: controlled trial of systematic one-stage screening in pregnancy', *The Lancet,* Vol.336, pp.387-391.

Thacker, S.B. (1985). 'Quality of controlled clinical trials. The case of imaging ultrasound in obstetrics: a review' *British Journal of Obstetric and Gynaecology,* Vol.92, pp.437-444.

CHAPTER NINE

Assessing the Effect of a New Health Technology

Rosemary Jenkins was a practising midwife, midwife teacher, midwifery manager before joining the Royal College of Midwives. Before leaving the RCM in 1994 she publicly challenged the stand taken by the RCOG on water births, as their attitude to it was not based on scientific fact. She feels equally strongly that the attitudes of midwives and women should also be based upon evidence.

Before I start on the subject matter of my paper, I'd like to tell you how I got here. It certainly wasn't because I am a passionate advocate of water birth. I'm sure if I were having a baby today, it's the last thing I would choose. I may want to lie in a bath to ease an aching back but it would end there. However, although not a water birth disciple, I have always felt strongly that women should have more choice about their care when having a baby and anything that might enable a wider range of choice should be seriously considered. But even that isn't why I'm here today. It's because I publicly challenged some obstetricians over horror stories on television, based on the flimsiest of evidence. I did a couple of broadcasts and got my only letter ever into the BMJ. And I thought that was it. Until Sheila Kitzinger rang me and asked me to speak at this conference and put the case particularly for more research. Looking at the programme there is a commendable amount already, but I hope to add some alternative thoughts.

I decided to discuss the same issues that I had taken up in the media, but on this occasion throw the same challenges and perhaps offer some solutions to you, the advocates rather than the antagonists of water birth. You see it is as wrong to introduce a new technology without assessment as it is to oppose its introduction without firm grounds.

A new technology you ask? We are talking about water birth. That's not technology, its a natural, non-interventionist approach to normal delivery. First I will argue that water birth should be considered a new technology; it should be assessed in the same way as other technologies and decisions on whether to make it universally available should be related to those assessments.

Is water birth a 'health technology'?

In 1992 the Department of Health in England published a paper, 'Assessing the Effects of Health Technologies'. In it, it said this:

> 'In this Report, we have taken the term "health technologies" to include all the methods used by health professionals to promote health, to prevent and treat disease, and to improve rehabilitation and long-term care. These methods include "hardware" such as syringes, medicines and high technology diagnostic imaging equipment; "software" such as education, diagnostic and therapeutic policies; as well as the skills and time of people working the health services.'

This is an extremely broad definition which, by including health promotion and therapeutic policies, includes in my view water birth. Indeed it also includes the development of the additional skills that health professionals need to assist at a water birth.

Although I hope that this contention - that water birth is a health technology - will generate some debate later this morning, the rest of my paper is based on an acceptance that it is and that it needs to be assessed as such.

The purpose of health technology assessment

There are some obvious reasons for assessing innovations in health care:

- Is the new treatment or management protocol safe?
- Does it do what it is supposed to do?
- Is it acceptable to the recipient?
- Is it acceptable to the clinician?

But there are two other questions that an evaluation should answer:

- How much does it cost?
- If the service spends money on this new development, what other service is not being offered?

All of these combine to raise the overriding question that health technology assessment sets out to answer.

Should this new development be made available and if it should, under what circumstances. Should it be:

- Freely available within the established state health care system;
- Available in a state system only if funding can be found;
- Available only through fee based systems or
- Not available at all.

Health technology assessment is above all a tool to assist policy and management decision making based upon evidence of safety, acceptability, effectiveness and efficiency.

That is one of the reasons why I felt so strongly about the misinformation being given out over the British media on the dangers of water birth based on a handful of cases. It was likely to result in hurried and ill thought out management decisions which would help no one, neither women nor the professionals looking after them. In retrospect we in this country know that to be true as some of maternity units started banning water birth even when women were choosing to have them in their own homes. But it is also the reason why the supporters of water birth should operate under the same constraints – that it will not be introduced unless and until we have more information about its effectiveness, efficiency and appropriateness.

The processes of assessment

From my comments on the need to guide management as well as clinical decisions you may have gathered that I am not just going to extol the virtues of the randomized controlled trial as the gold standard assessment tool, but discuss other forms of evaluation that must be conducted. In fact when I return later to the randomized controlled trial I am going to offer some healthy scepticism about it.

Before looking at the clinical implications of water birth, I want to argue for economic studies of the potential impact of water birth within a large health care system like the UK NHS. So far in this conference the presentations have not touched upon this aspect of this new technology. But there is a cost to water birth.

There are of course the installation costs of the pools themselves. But there is the opportunity cost of using rooms that could be used for other purposes. There is the cost of staff training and again the additional opportunity cost of what is lost while that training takes place. What would a midwife be doing if she weren't on a training course or what other skill could she be learning if she were not learning how to assist at a water birth? We have to examine the economic cost of water birth because any resources spent on one activity represent a failure to put those resources somewhere else. We need to be quite certain that energy, skills and money are being directed towards producing optimal outcomes.

In the context of a whole health care system, this might even mean that the introduction of water birth on a widespread scale could displace an increased service to the mentally ill, the chronically disabled or intensive care beds. Maternity services cannot be divorced from the rest of the health service.

This is not necessarily an argument against making water birth widely available thus increasing the range of choice for women. Rather it is a plea that an assessment of its potential economic cost should be compared with alternative uses for resources; it is a plea that if water birth is made available, the decision to do this has been rationally made based upon the whole cost – actual costs and opportunity costs of the intervention.

It is a plea that if introduced it is because it is the most efficient way to use the available resources and that it will not introduce inequity into the system by giving greater choice to one group and the expense of choice for another group of health service users.

Researching safety

No amount of economic analysis will justify the inclusion of a new intervention if that intervention is shown to be unsafe. There are a number of methods for examining the possible impact of water birth, and the papers in this conference show that many of these are currently in use. All of them however have limitation and the subject matter – water birth – can exacerbate these. I want to touch on some of the difficulties that some of these methods can encounter and then discuss a relatively new form of trial that might be appropriate.

Research into water birth can present three major problems for the researchers. First it is the problem of numbers, second the problem of choice of variables and third the problem of bias.

One of the aims of clinical research is to show the effect of a treatment and prove that the effect did not happen by chance. A study needs sufficient subjects so that when the results are analysed the researchers can be confident that the results achieve statistical significance. If studies are small, you will have to wait until sufficient are done to allow meta analysis to reveal their significance. Equally, observational studies may have to draw upon subjects from many centres or over a long time span to have sufficient numbers to make any conclusions convincing. But there aren't many water births.

Secondly, there is the problem of what to test for. The report of the NPEU suggested a number of areas for research, some of them about the management of the technique itself. But what about comparative studies? What to use to compare with other forms of birth? What variables are common enough to yield sufficient data when water birth uptake remains small? Certainly not perinatal mortality in western developed countries. Yet this is the one issue that influences the public, the media and the sceptical professions. It is probable that for all their limitations, the impact of water birth on perinatal mortality will probably need to be drawn from observational and analytical studies rather than from the gold standard randomized controlled trial. If its any consolation, the link between smoking and lung cancer was never proven with an randomized controlled trial but by a raft of well designed epidemiological studies. But unlike water birth and perinatal loss, the smoking/lung cancer link is very strong and smoking common. I predict, therefore, that it will probably never be possible to ward off the dyed-in-the-wool critic who uses the perinatal loss argument to frustrate an expansion of birth in water. Research is however, likely to give answers for more common variables - infection, caesarean section rates, forceps and satisfaction levels. You will have to rely on a package of positive results for those variables to offset the negative effect of even a single reported baby death as a direct result of being born in a bath. It is a conundrum that the researchers may take some time to solve.

Thirdly, there is the problem of bias. Bias is a systematic error in a study which results in an incorrect estimate of the association between exposure (in this case the water birth itself) and disease (for example, morbidity and mortality associated with birth in water). It can create problems, particularly in retrospective observational studies and in case-control studies but it is commonly accepted that a properly designed randomized control trial eliminates this difficulty. I don't believe that this is entirely true in the particular circumstance of water birth.

In a randomized controlled trial, subjects who agree to participate are then randomly assigned to a treatment and a non-treatment group. Because of this randomization the accepted wisdom is that potential biases are eliminated and any differences between the study group and the controls can therefore be attributed solely to the effect of the intervention. As long as the numbers in the study are large enough to achieve statistical significance when the data are analysed, the results should be accepted with some confidence - an unbiased study. But there can be a source of bias in an randomized controlled trial and I believe that this can be quite significant in water birth. There is a choice made in randomized controlled trials which is not random and that is a choice to enter the trial or not.

Water birth is not everyone's choice. I said at the beginning that it would not be mine. If I were confronted with a request to enter a trial of water birth and be randomly assigned to either an in-pool or an out of pool group, I am unlikely to agree to participate. Equally, if I am a woman who is set upon having a water birth, I would not want to risk not having it. I would also be unlikely to enter the trial. The only women who would want to consent to the research are those who have no preference either way. The big question that then needs to be resolved is, are these two groups, those who chose to exercise a preference and those who do not, different. If they are, this may be a fundamental source of bias.

This problem with the randomized controlled trial has been recognized for some time. Brewin and Bradley, writing in the BMJ in 1989 said;

> 'Allocating patients to treatment in a systematic non-randomized way may introduce bias which destroys comparability. We argue here that despite this advantage random allocation is not always suitable. Though patients play an active part in the outcome of all treatments, we suggest that clinical trials in which they are required to sustain an effortful and demanding role and those in which they are likely to have strong preferences for one treatment need to be considered differently.'

This could not describe the birth in water situation better. They went on to describe preference trials. This type of clinical trial has now also been used in breast cancer treatments and treatment for prostatic hypertrophy.

The preference trial aims to combine a randomized trial alongside a trial where preferences for treatment are allowed.

There are two major arms to the trial. Those who have a preference for their treatment, whether that is to have the treatment or not, and those with no preference who are randomized as in any randomized controlled trial. There will then be four groups whose outcomes can be compared, the randomly allocated treatment and non treatment groups and the preference treated and non treated groups. Additionally however, the whole group that agreed to randomization can be compared with the group who followed their preferences to see whether there are differences of importance between these two.

I think we may see much more of this type of research over a whole range of treatments as patients are involved more in the decision making processes and may wish to exercise greater personal preference over what happens to them even when participating in research. I believe it offers one of the most appropriate study designs for birth in water. After all, to reiterate the words of Brewin, this is a group of women who sustain an effortful and demanding role in the treatment and are likely to have strong preferences.

Conclusion

I have argued in my paper for water birth to be considered along with all other health technologies, to be subjected to economic analysis and clinical trial before it becomes widely disseminated in the health care system. This is not to stop it or to give it a green light. Rather it is to enable a rational decision to be made based on rational evaluation. If it is proven effective, safe and efficient, then we can be confident that the choice can be extended widely to all women. If not then we should be just as confident in a decision not to invest time, skills, space and energy into extending its provision.

PART FIVE

Water Birth and the Midwife

CHAPTER TEN

Water Birth and the Role of the Midwife

Caroline Flint is a registered midwife in practice with The Birth Centre Ltd. This is a small practice of independent midwives who do many home births and opened the UK's first Birth Centre in June 1994. Each Birthroom has its own Birthing Pool - the Centre is in South London and is used by women from all over the South of England. Caroline is President of the Royal College of Midwives and Honorary Professor Thames Valley University. She has written four books on midwifery and over 250 articles. Caroline has been a midwife for nearly 20 years, and a National Childbirth Trust teacher for 25 years.

For the midwife, water birth is an exciting and interesting addition to normal practice. It appears to give women enormous pain relief during labour and enables the woman to be more buoyant and mobile during the labour. For the midwife it is easy to look after a woman in water because she has a full view of the whole woman, she can see what is going on.

When midwives first attend water births they are often anxious, but the way they think and feel about birth and their relationship with the woman starts to change in a positive way - and with it, their practice.

In some ways, what midwives learn from their experience of water births shows them how to give better help to women in all labours.

Looking after women in labour in water, and giving birth in water, is an important way of training midwives to develop new skills and to support the natural process, it reinforces the supportive and enabling role of the midwife compared with trying to 'manage' birth in the way that the obstetric process does. A woman in a pool is in her own space. She is in charge. She is inviolate. Midwives have to think carefully before intruding. It probably reduces interventions which can be unnecessary and sometimes even harmful.

Because of the buoyancy provided by water, a woman can move easily and spontaneously frequently changing her position. Midwives are already aware of how rocking, rotating and slanting the pelvis, crouching and floating and being on all fours not only eases the pain, but can facilitate rotation and descent of the fetal head. With water birth and labour this is strongly apparent - being with women around water can be a transforming experience for midwives.

Thoughts

The first water birth a midwife attends can make her quite nervous. She knows in theory that the birth will progress like any other birth but she is not quite sure how she should behave, will she be able to gauge the progress of the labour? Will she be expected to get into the water? What if something goes wrong - how will she get the woman out of the water?

How will she judge the amount of the blood loss? How will she guard the perineum or for that matter how will she cut an episiotomy if it is necessary? If she has not got a specially adapted sonic aid, how will she listen to the fetal heart? What if the cord is around the baby's neck - how will she cope?

The midwife reads everything she can on water birth, she goes to a Study Day if possible, she watches a video on water birth and waits with some nervousness for the call.

Feelings

No-one likes to feel insecure, midwives least of all. The midwifery profession has a very high level of scrutiny of each midwife's practice by Supervisors of Midwives. If a midwife gets something wrong she is aware that the penalties are severe, two lives are in her hands and her feelings of responsibilities are great.

The midwife fears that she won't be able to manage, that something may go wrong, not enough research has been done into water births and she doesn't want to harm either mother or baby. She recalls the media furore over water births a couple of years ago, she asks her Supervisor for assistance - the response is to make sure the water does not overheat the mother and baby. She asks the woman if she has a thermometer - usually this comes with the pool.

Practice

The practice of the midwife is also influenced when a woman decides on a water birth. Firstly the balance of power is affected by the fact that the woman is cocooned in a watery tub, inaccessible unless she decides that she wants to be. The number of women, who when I have said to them 'Can I listen to the baby's heart please' have just moved to the far side of the tub and said firmly 'No' is legion! I well remember the woman who when I put my gloved hand out to catch her baby just propelled herself to the far side of the pool and delivered her baby herself. When the woman is in the pool she is in charge, she is more mobile than she has been, thanks to the buoyancy of the water, she is inviolate because no one else is likely to come inside the pool with her, she is more powerful because the water seems to help the pain so much.

With the right equipment the midwife can monitor the baby's heart beat without needing the woman to emerge from the water. An underwater sonicaid is indispensable. The woman will look after herself in the pool, only needing encouraging words and drinks.

The arrival of the baby is usually effected very smoothly, I usually bring the baby to the surface immediately but I know others may have a theory that the baby will not breathe whilst it is underwater - a theory I am too nervous to test! Often the woman gets out for the third stage - but equally often doesn't, the placenta emerges eventually.

Clearing up after a water birth is easily achieved by just pulling the plug or by asking the woman to emerge from the water and then someone else pumps out the water from the pool. The midwife's role is an extremely practical one, she needs to protect the floor from drips of either water or blood and she needs to ensure the safety of both mother and baby.

Water birth - the effect on midwives

Labouring in water gives a woman greater privacy because the midwife does not have access to the woman unless the woman specifically gives the midwife that access. The issues of power and control are affected by a woman having a water birth and the midwife is in a more subservient situation than she is normally. Because women are more mobile in water and also because the water is somewhat soiled, midwives do not normally get into the water with the woman.

Babies born in water appear to remain a purple colour for longer than babies born into air, and this can be worrying for the midwife, and if the baby needs some resuscitation it can be difficult and a bit slippery trying to clamp and cut the cord in order to get the baby to the resuscitaire.

For the midwife there is very little clearing up after the delivery which is a bonus for her and the huge amount of pain relief it appears to give women is such a bonus that it is a lovely easy way of looking after women and it's exciting to have such variety in one's work.

CHAPTER ELEVEN

Water and Pain Relief – Observations of Over 570 Births at Hillingdon

> **Cass Nightingale** has been a midwife since 1967 and a manager since 1978, she is now Divisional Manager of Women's and Children's Services at Hillingdon Hospital, London. She has maintained her clinical skills, and has a special interest in the use of water in labour and in water birth. This interest developed whilst working at Hinchingbrook Hospital Huntingdon, following a visit to Pithivier, France. As a Supervisor of Midwives she feels it is extremely important that midwives are adequately trained to carry out water births and are aware of the possible emergencies, and how to deal with them should they arise.

Hillingdon Hospital has had the benefit of a large bath and five ordinary baths within the Labour Ward area since June 1990.

Initially, it was envisaged that water would be offered for relaxation and pain relief. In September of that year, however, we delivered our first baby in water, to a lady who found the water so relaxing that she refused to get out.

The lady was a primip and the baby weighed eight and a half pounds, the perineum was intact. Little did she know at the time just how much this birth was to change practice at Hillingdon - she has since gone on to have a further two water births.

In 1994 there were 3,505 births at Hillingdon, 74 per cent of these were spontaneous vaginal deliveries.

Sixty per cent of women admitted to the Unit used water at sometime during their labour, five per cent of the normal births were in water (three and a half per cent of all births).

Initially both midwives and medical staff were very sceptical regarding the pain relieving properties of something as simple as water.

In the year running up to the opening of the new labour ward a considerable amount of in-service training was organized, covering many subjects including mobilization in labour, the use of water, and emergency delivery in water.

It should be stressed to any midwife, caring for women in water as a method of pain relief, that she must be prepared to deliver in water. Often women progress rapidly and are unable to get out of the bath, and sometimes women just find the effects of using water so relaxing they just do not want to get out.

Some staff spent a few days at Hinchingbrooke Hospital, in Huntingdon, observing natural births and the use of water for pain relief.

Most came back fired with enthusiasm, but had some doubts as to how this type of care could be offered in a much busier Unit.

In actual fact, water very quickly became our first method of pain relief.

Unfortunately we have never kept statistics of women using the water solely for pain relief in labour, but I would estimate that between 50-60 per cent of women delivering at Hillingdon use water at some time during their labour.

Why does water ease pain?

Physiologically, endorphins are released to ease the painful contractions.

However, when admitted in labour most women are anxious, and anxiety produces adrenaline. This inhibits the effect of the endorphins, causing women to become tense, and preventing labour progressing despite painful contractions.

The offer of a warm relaxing bath, something which is familiar to all of us, greatly aids relaxation enabling labour to progress as it should.

At Hillingdon the Birthing Room with the large bathroom attached is situated at the quietest part of the labour ward, away from the hustle and bustle of the main corridors.

It is a peaceful, secure, environment where both woman and midwife can be left alone to get on with labour.

Most women relax very quickly and become less tense, they are more buoyant and thus are able to move about more freely.

To date the bath has provided excellent pain relief for several women who have had severe back problems, and one who developed a split symphysis nearing the end of her pregnancy.

Most women will sleep between contractions within 10-15 minutes of entering the bath.

Usage of water

In early labour

Water is used in early labour to ease backache, relieve tension, and to enhance relaxation.

As we only have one large bath the smaller baths are generally used at this time. The women find them easy to get in and out of, and they can more easily combine mobilization with relaxation in water.

When labour is well established and the cervix has dilated to 4-5 centimetres, deep water reduces pain and enables the women to relax in comfort. This is usually when they start to use the big bath.

Although the contractions often appear to be shorter in length and less frequent, dilatation of the cervix is usually more rapid in water.

In 1994 one of our BSc. midwifery students, as part of her dissertation, looked at and compared the labours of 101 women delivering in water and a similar group delivering out of water (Table 11.1).

Sample		
WATERBIRTH	**Ist stage**	**5.53**
	2nd stage	**1.34**
	Total	**7.27 mins**
CONTROL (BED)	**Ist stage**	**9.29**
	2nd stage	**0.34**
	Total	**10.03**

Table 11.1: Comparison of labours in and out of water

We feel that the longer second stage in the water birth group is possibly due to the fact that women in water are not actively encouraged to push with each contraction as not all contractions are expulsive in nature. The women are very much advised to do what their body tells them.

For delivery

It is very unusual for women to use water solely for delivery, the great majority use it initially for pain relief and relaxation and then go on to deliver in it.

We are very happy for women to use Entonox (50 per cent oxygen and 50 per cent Nitrous Oxide) to aid pain relief in the water. However, it is our experience that they tend to use it just before entering the pool, but as the water takes effect they no longer require it.

Some women request the Entonox again just at the end of the first stage of labour and again discard it once they start to push.

We tend to find that if the water is going to be an effective method of pain relief it works within 10-15 minutes.

In our experience, where water is not effective women tend to opt for epidural anaesthesia.

As mentioned earlier, contractions are not always expulsive in the second stage. Women use their contractions best when they want to push.

The tissues of the vulva and perineum are softened by the warm water and appear to stretch more easily.

Of the 570 births in water, just seven women have required an episiotomy. Five of these required no local analgesia, two stood up whilst the perineum was infiltrated with lignocaine.

Most women experience less perineal pain in water, therefore the delivery is more controlled.

CLIENT PREPARATION

It is *not* essential for women and their partners to attend a class on water birth but one is held every Wednesday evening.

Those that attend are told the advantages and disadvantages of the use of water.

Advantages:
- As the bath is plumbed in at Hillingdon it is easy to use.
- It is non-invasive.
- It does not appear detrimental to the baby at all.
- It is relaxing.
- It offers good pain relief.
- Women remain in control of their labour.
- Women can always go on to other analgesia.

Disadvantages:
- The room tends to be very warm.
- The bath can be restrictive.
- The fetal heart rate cannot be continuously monitored.
- It can slow down the labour if used too early.
- It does not always work.
- At present it is only available for normal low risk labour e.g. cephalic presentations of at least 37 weeks gestation.

It is important for couples to realize that when they are opting for a water birth they are also opting for a drug free labour. However, they should be reassured that other analgesia is available should it be required.

They are informed of our current statistics, e.g. number of water births and outcomes. They are shown a video. A visit is made to the Labour Ward and pool room. Self help tips are given, e.g. they are advised to practice sitting crossed legged on the floor to help stretch the thigh muscles, to practice squatting holding on to the back of a chair, to practice squatting with their partner supporting them, and finally to do some gentle arm exercises. If they go home and do these, most women are able to support themselves in the bath which prevents damage to the midwife's back!

We also have Yoga/active birth classes available.

It is important that couples are given *all* the information to enable them to make a decision on the type of birth they wish to have.

The realities are, that of perhaps 12 couples attending a class just 25 per cent will have a water birth, around 50 per cent will use water just for pain relief, and the remaining 25 per cent will not use water at all.

Whilst on the subject of pain I feel it is important to mention the midwife's back! We fortunately have not had any problems with back injuries.

Comfortable stools are provided in the bathroom for midwives to sit on, this enables them to have eye to eye contact with the women, and to listen to the fetal heart rate without bending.

Women basically deliver themselves, and therefore the midwife should only need to lean over the bath on one or two occasions - to feel for the umbilical cord around the baby's neck, and to lift the baby out of the water.

Finally, I would like to emphasise the skills of the midwife, it is important that women are cared for by midwives who are confident in their ability to support women who want a drug free labour, and who choose to use water for either pain relief, or to deliver in.

Both women and midwives should feel supported at *all* times, and it is only by ensuring this, that we can extend the use of water so that *all* women can have the benefit of good pain relief which is not at all invasive.

Results

September 1990 - March 1995

Primigravidae	248	(43.5%)
Multigravidae	322	(56.5%)

Perineal damage

	Primips	Multips
Intact Perineum	88 (35%)	169 (52%)
Ist degree tear	23	75
2nd degree tear	129	75
3rd degree tear	1	3
Episiotomy	7	0
	248	322

Figures rounded off

Overall suture rate 1994 = 26 per cent

Blood loss

Estimated blood loss	Number	Percentage (%)
0 - 500mls	541	95
501 - 1000mls	27	4.7
1001 - 1500mls	2	0.3
	570	100

Figures rounded off

Three women required blood transfusion.

Apgar at 1 minute	No. of babies	Percentage (%)
8>	520	91
7	30	5
6	13	2.2
5	4	0.7
4	3	0.53
	570	100

Figures rounded off

Table 11.2: The Hillington Hospital Water Birth Statistics

Admissions to neonatal unit immediately post delivery

1. Apgar 4 Hypoxic (No reason found) Ventilated + antibiotics.
2. Apgar 8 Meconium. Aspiration.
3. Apgar 8 Grunting respirations at one hour - 12 hours observation only.
4. Apgar 9 Grunty respirations at one hour - 12 hours observation only.
5. Apgar 9 Mucosy ++ Oesophageal Atresia with Fistula (operated on at Great Ormond Street).

All babies made a good recovery.

Admitted between 4th and 7th day
- 2 with urinary tract infection.
- 2 with an infected cord (Day 7).
- 1 Jaundiced and dehydrated (Day 7) Feeding problems.

It has been interesting to note that the incidence of suturing has declined with the advent of water births. Many of the second degree tears are small and medial, and the midwives have the confidence to allow them to heal without suturing, which appears to be far more comfortable for the women.

The episiotomy rate is very low and is only performed as a last resort.

Blood loss is purely a guestimate but it is worth noting that the postpartum haemorrhage rate has gradually declined as midwives have become used to dealing with a physiological third stage.

The results for the babies are fairly self explanatory, the first baby with an Apgar score of four cried instantly once brought to the surface, but then went flat and required resuscitation. No real explanation was found, but he required ventilation and antibiotics for around 48 hours post delivery.

The second baby was born in good condition but inhaled meconium, which was only apparent as the anterior shoulder was delivered.

He too was ventilated and treated with antibiotics, he also had a hare lip, cleft palate and hyperspadias.

The next two babies were born in good condition but were noted to have slightly grunting respirations at one to one and a half hours of age. They were admitted to the Neonatal Unit for observation but required no treatment.

The last baby was born in good condition but noted to be very mucosy, she was diagnosed as having a tracheo-oesophageal fistula, which was later repaired.

All the babies made a good recovery.

CHAPTER TWELVE

The Role of the Midwifery Supervisor

Dianne Garland is the Senior Midwife in Practice and Research Development at Maidstone Hospital, Kent. She has been a practising midwife for twelve years, eleven of those at Maidstone. During this time she's worked in clinical, education, and managerial roles. Since 1987 she has undertaken many water births in her role as midwife and supervisor, and has established a network of colleagues in the south east. She travels, writes and lectures widely both in the UK and abroad, including America and Japan. In conjunction with local companies she designed a water birthing tub, and the first underwater fetal heart rate doppler.

Supervision of Midwives has been written into UK statute since 1902 and despite several Acts (1936, 1951 and 1974) this statutory obligation has basically remained unchanged. It is still beholden on Supervisors to maintain identified set objectives:

- To set standards
- To ensure competent practitioners
- To support staff who are having difficulties
- Identification of continuing training needs
- Protection of the public

Changes to the Local Supervising Authority (LAS) are before Parliament in the Health Authorities Bill which will come into force April 1996. This will transfer the function of LAS to the new Health Authorities (mergers between old DHA and the Family Health Services Authority).

As Supervisors of Midwives we are appointed to be advocates for clients and supporters to midwives. This role seemed to be reflected well in the area of water labour/birth and can be related to the eleven letters of the word *supervision*.

S - Support

I aim to provide both physical and psychological support to midwives and parents wishing to use water for labour and/or delivery. I interview all staff and clients who may be interested in this type of care and support them in their choices and clinical decisions.

As part of this support I have involved other specialists if the clinical situation is on the fringes of normality. Many clients have asked to use water for labour or delivery, when they have had a previous caesarean section. At the present time we do not offer this facility for these women so, as Supervisor, I discuss the reasons why and offer support as they decide upon another option.

U - Unbiased

This should be seen truly to reflect current knowledge and information. I share all the recorded advantages and disadvantages with parents and staff. I do not believe in hiding or failing to give true accounts of the pitfalls that I have encountered over the last seven years.

Midwives often voice concerns over legal and professional accountability surrounding water births. Cases that have come to light over the past few years have highlighted just how vulnerable some midwives feel.

When I talk to women I discuss the experiences we have had at Maidstone, and when problems have occurred how we deal with them both practically and physiologically.

P - Parameters

Parameters for practice should reflect clinical knowledge and expertise. These parameters could then act as guidelines for practice in both hospital and community settings, and can be shared with parents as a marker for current knowledge base.

The guidelines that we have designed at Maidstone are reviewed regularly between clinicians, managers and supervisors. We alter them as we gain new clinical experience or in light of research evidence. They are widely available to women and midwives through the Maternity Unit. Over the past seven years, as Supervisor, I have shared them with other units who often use them as a foundation to their own parameters for practice.

E - Education

Education is a role that as Supervisors we should be seen to be encouraging. The Midwives Code of Practice states that 'we should receive adequate preparation and training in new skills'. Supervisors have, I believe, an important role in facilitating this education so midwives feel prepared to take on this water birth role.

Part of this education is to offer three monthly updates to my own midwives. We run these at different times through the day so that all staff have access to the sessions. A large data base is available in the Maternity Unit and, as Supervisor, I keep a separate notice board up to date on the labour ward.

I offer bi-monthly water birth parentcraft sessions for interested parents. At these sessions we discuss the practical issues of using water for labour and delivery and the experiences of 500 water births at Maidstone.

R - Resource and learning opportunities

As Supervisors it is vital that we act as a resource for learning materials and clinical experiences. If we are unable to offer these opportunities, then we should facilitate midwives to seek out this type of experience and colleagues who can skill share.

Part of this resource sharing is to offer clinical experience at Maidstone. We cannot guarantee that colleagues will always see a water birth. We share our experiences and the vast amount of data we have, whilst our midwives share their own clinical cases with visitors.

As a Supervisor I have also acted as a resource to a variety of organizations, including the Royal College of Midwives and National Perinatal Epidemiology Unit.

V - Visionaries

Visionaries for our profession in clinical and managerial area. I believe that Supervisors should be seen as leading the profession forward and assist midwives who are expanding the parameters of care and knowledge.

This means that as supervisors we must heed current trends and service changes. Being aware of these changes and how, if appropriate, we can alter practice or adapt to take on board new clinical care. Inherent within this is the need to review care and facilitate this change with staff and act as a change agent.

I - Integrity: with parents and colleagues

We need to be seen as impartial and open with all those involved. Encouraging others to network increases this integrity and this conference is a prime example.

Here we can see how many practitioners are currently working on water births. As Supervisor, this networking has led to many opportunities to lecture abroad. This skill sharing across the ocean has developed into a unique bond between American and UK midwives. As time goes on, and with this type of conference, this professional integrity can then be shared with colleagues and parents.

S - Structure

Structure involving a liaison role for Supervisors to organize the clinical and theoretical aspects of practice. Organizational structure in today's NHS means including non midwifery managers and clinical directors, so that they are aware of the role of the midwives in water births.

This type of structural support can pay dividends. In my capacity as Supervisor I liaise with many other health professionals, doctors, midwives, health visitors and infection control nurses. In seven years of water birthing practice, the opportunity to utilize this structure between peer to peer had proved invaluable.

I - Investigation

We are charged as Supervisors to investigate any clinical issue of concern. It is vital that midwives maintain complete records, and, contained within these, specific notes of water temperature and monitoring of mother and baby. These records also assist if any investigatory procedure is necessary.

This investigation also includes reviewing practice in light of new or controversial evidence. Following the issues of hypothermia in 1993, the Maternity Unit reviewed their water temperature policy. As Supervisor it was my role to investigate if there was a need to alter our labour water temperatures. Following our review, it was felt unnecessary to alter our practice.

O - Observation

Observation of water births by Supervisors can assist us in being more able to 'judge' and comment on practice. If we have seen and preferably undertaken a water birth, it is much easier to comment on practice and utilize the Bolum test. That is as midwives we are 'judged' on the practice accepted as standard by our peers.

Observation at Maidstone is offered to all staff who practice within the Department. Staff who wish to observe water births include midwives and doctors, and do so once the mother's permission has been sought. This acts as a skill sharing and learning opportunity.

N - Nurturing

An old fashioned word but one that I believe sums up my view of Supervision. In its literal sense it means 'bringing up' and 'care'. As a Supervisor this is fundamental to my practice.

I care for, and about, the midwives with whom I work. This nurturing is fostered through my role as Supervisor, as I work clinically with my colleagues when undertaking water births.

This nurturing assists midwives to a level whereby they can take over this role themselves. As a Supervisor, I nurture parents to expand their own knowledge and thus make an informed choice regarding the use of water for labour and delivery.

I would like to finish by sharing two short clinical scenarios where I have utilized Supervision and I have played a role in fostering a supportive environment.

Clinical scenario - supervision

I was involved in a clinical case where it would be the first time that a previous caesarean section client was to have a water birth.

Time was spent talking and planning between the Consultant, Community Midwife and Supervisor. This multi disciplinary approach included Michelle who spoke about her wish to have a water birth with her second child, but this had not been possible within the Unit's criteria. With her third pregnancy she again spoke to her Community Midwife about this option.

As Supervisor, I was involved both in clinical and professional support. A joint decision was made that a rota between the Community Midwife and two Supervisors would exist. In this way Michelle knew that one of these three would deliver her.

A trusting and supportive environment was fostered, with Michelle gaining confidence from this system. For the midwives it provided an opportunity to utilize the Supervisors in their true professional role.

The water birth was a great success and no problems occurred. I was on call the night Michelle went into labour. After a smooth and short labour, a gentle birth occurred with the delivery of a baby girl.

Supervision scenario

Karen was both a friend and colleague. Although she was not a midwife we had worked closely together in the hospital for many years. When she found herself pregnant with her second child it seemed the most natural thing to ask her friend, me, to deliver her.

Karen's first labour and delivery had been three years earlier in another hospital. The labour was induced, long and compounded by hormonal intravenous stimulation, epidural and episiotomy. Her son was born vaginally but her birth experience was marred by memories of intervention, slow postnatal recovery and the need to have the episiotomy resutured.

Added to this, Karen suffers from Multiple Sclerosis but was at the time of booking in remission.

Karen and I spoke early in her pregnancy about using water for labour and, if all was going well, that she would like to stay in and deliver. I went to Karen's home at 35 weeks to discuss with her, Kevin her partner and a very inquisitive three year old, just what was involved in using the tubs.

We had already involved her Consultant who had no problem with Karen using the tub, so long as her MS was still in remission.

Karen said that she felt her previous labour was 'controlled' by the health professionals and she was so weary during labour, particularly as she was not permitted to eat or drink.

As you will probably have gathered, I was keen to provide a very different birth experience for Karen and her family. I had high expectations of myself but felt it was vital as Supervisor to, as it was, 'put my money where my mouth is', and care for Karen.

Labour and delivery went without a hitch. A short labour, rapid water birth and the delightful birth of a 9lb 1oz baby girl. (Incidentally, a small tear was the only perineal damage).

As Supervisor it reminded me how important clinical hands on work remains. And as a friend it was a wonderful experience.

Further reading

English National Board (1992). *Preparation for Supervisors of Midwives.* London: ENB.

Garland, D. (1995). *Waterbirth - An Attitude to Care.* Hale, Cheshire: Books for Midwives Press.

Harmond, K. (1995). 'Devolving supervision', *Modern Midwife,* Vol.5, No.10, October pp.18-21.

PART SIX

Water Birth and the Obstetrician

CHAPTER THIRTEEN

A Thousand Water Births: Selection Criteria and Outcome

> **Josie Muscat** runs one of the most modern private clinics in Malta and in 1988 established Malta's first Underwater Childbirth Clinic. It has achieved one of the highest international rates of underwater births per head of population. Dr Muscat is married to Franca Camilleri, has six children, one of whom has Down's Syndrome. This led Dr Muscat to set up the Eden Foundation, a non-profit organization dedicated to the education of mentally disadvantaged children, with the aim of integrating them in the community and helping them achieve independence.

A pregnant mother enters my office and asks,

> 'Can I deliver my baby under water? Is it safe? Could you tell me more about it? Can my baby drown? Will my baby swallow water?'

Obviously what parents-to-be are after is concrete proof that water birth is something not only worth trying but that it is completely safe for both the mother and baby.

Citing what today is accepted as the norm for water births – relaxation, weightlessness, cleanliness, privacy, less likelihood of a tear – does not always get the message through since people and professionals ask for facts and statistics rather than statements. Considering that water births is an innovative method of delivery, parents are told all sorts of sensationalist statements. What impresses is what is said by people who have no experience at all in this field.

The selective criteria and outcome of the first consecutive 1000 water births carried out at the St. James Birth Centre might serve as a basis for further research and a guide to those who would like to venture into this alternative method. Attempts were made to compare the outcome with a similar number of traditional deliveries or dry births but it was soon realized that it was difficult to compare the two populations.

At the St. James Birth Centre we have no pre-conceived rules. Time is not a factor. Since we do not have Special Care Baby Unit (SCBU) facilities, we do not accept high risk cases such as severe Intra-Uterine Growth Retardation (IUGR); or babies expected to be below 2.5 kilograms or if they go into labour before 36 weeks gestation; mothers with placenta praevia; multiple pregnancies of triplets and over; diabetics on insulin; severe pregnancy induced hypertension; and known cases of fetal anomalies. But we do accept breech deliveries; twin pregnancy, mild hypertension; previous caesarean section.

We have never tried breech and twin deliveries in water. We feel that in such cases quick decisions might have to be taken and moving the mother out of the water might complicate matters with loss of valuable time. But mothers can make use of the bath and pool facilities up to the end of the first stage of labour. They are then asked to leave the bath and delivery is carried out in the traditional method.

Initial anecdotal results have shown that mothers with slight hypertension (150/90 not more) seem to benefit from the relaxation of warm water, quiet surroundings, light music, sounds of water and the presence and reassurance of the Childbirth Educator, whom she has known all through her pregnancy and who gives all the necessary support and encouragement. Mothers who opt for a water delivery are free to choose between staying in a pool during the first stage and then moving into a special compartment with an inbuilt birthing chair to deliver, or going for a second option only.

All our mothers are followed up antenatally by myself and they are finally scanned at 38 weeks gestation to measure the size of the head (biparietal diameter - BPD) and the expected birth weight. These two biometric measurements, together with the height and shoe size, indicate whether special precautions are necessary and whether we have to be on our guard for cephalo-pelvic disproportion (CPD) or a difficult delivery. A standing lateral pelvimetry is only resorted to in rare cases since we believe that best pelvimetry is labour itself.

We do not induce labour, unless the mother is past 41 weeks gestation and even then we try to avoid drugs as much as possible. We give great importance to Manning's score (bio physical profile where the mother is past 40 weeks gestation).

In the case of a favourable cervix (almost fully effaced; soft and maybe even one centimetre dilated) we prefer to administer 50ml of castor oil mixed with six squeezed oranges and one tablespoon of sugar. In most cases this stimulates labour and saves us having to make use of prostaglandins or synthetic oxytocin or syntocinon drips.

In a few instances we find out that this stimulation fades out towards the end of labour and the administration of a small dose of oxytocin, of not more than one unit, might be necessary to stimulate effective final contractions. Should uterine atony set in or the mother is too tired to bear down, then an oxytocin infusion is set up. If there is arrested descent of the fetal head and a ventouse delivery is indicated then the following criteria is used:

If the head is at station 0 or less the mother is taken out of the water and ventouse delivery is carried out in the usual manner.

If the head is at station +1 or more, a rubber cup is applied with the mother still in the tub and the baby is delivered in water.

No episiotomies are ever done in water. If a tear ensues it is usually never more than a second degree tear requiring three or four stitches. Not a single fourth degree tear was recorded in water. In the case of a tear this is usually repaired under local anaesthesia in bed. We never had any complications from such tears.

Ergometrine maleate (syntometrine) is only given post partum if the mother has a prolonged labour due to a large baby (4.2 kilos or more); if she is very tired or needed an instrumental (ventouse) delivery; in the case of an atonic uterus; a past history of post partum haemorrhage, if the mother starts bleeding more than normally or if the fundus does not involute. Out of 1,000 births ergometrine was administered in only 44 cases (4.4 per cent).

The placenta is delivered with the mother still in the water. When the baby is born, at times we place one hand on the fundus, to help keep it contracted to avoid bleeding.

At the birth of the baby we start to empty the water to one third its original level better to observe undue bleeding. Once the placenta is delivered then the water is drained and the mother is given a shower and helped to her room. Should the mother feel faint or very tired, she can lie flat in the bath, she is given a cold shower and a sweet hot drink. Only in very rare cases do we have to resort to lifting the mother to her bed.

The 1000 mothers who made use of the bath to deliver satisfied the above mentioned criteria. Women are given the choice of choosing between a water or traditional delivery. No one is forced to use either. But we dissuade obese women from delivering in the bath.

No age limit is set; if an oxytocin infusion has been set up the mother is still allowed to enter the bath with the infusion in place. The fetal heart is monitored with a hand held fetal Doppler. The mother is free to leave the bath when and if she so decides.

She is encouraged to leave if she is too tired or if no progress in fetal descent is recorded. In very obese mothers or mothers with a pendulous abdomen we find that descent of the fetal head is assessed better in the supine position with a couple of pillows behind. The mother is encouraged to take up any position she feels comfortable in. She might be asked to change position if this helps in the progress of descent or the mother bears down better in such a position.

The number of babies transferred to the SCBU was five with one neonatal death due to severe meconium aspiration syndrome.

Water temperature

We go by no fixed temperature. It is the mother who decides what temperature she prefers. On average this varies between 33C° and 38C° no higher in the birthing bath. Mothers who make use of the pool in the first stage seem to prefer cooler temperatures. In fact on average, pool temperature varies between 28C° and 32C°.

The range of perception of pain using a visual analogue scale (slide rule) varies considerably by 10-90 per cent less, but on average pain perception in the bath is 50 per cent less.

I would like to emphasise that the outcome of the first 1000 water births is the result of team work, starting from the very first clinic visit the mother attends to two weeks following birth. The team consists of three midwives, two childbirth educators and myself.

Each mother is assigned a midwife and childbirth educator who follow her up antenatally, during labour and postnatally. There are no shifts or fixed hours of work and they get paid per mother they attend. All of us work happily together as a team. We respect each other's abilities and limitations, each of us has our individual, essential, role to play in the process of labour and delivery.

Apgar Score		
Apgar > 9 after 1 minute	982	98.2%
Apgar < 9 after 5 minutes	13	1.3%
Apgar < 9 after 10 minutes	5	0.5%
Neonatal Death	1	0.1%

1000 Water Births		
Primigravidae	488	48.8%
Multigravidae	512	51.2%

Syntometrine		
Syntometrine was used in 44 cases		4.40%

Augmentations		
Augmentation with Syntocinon	126	12.6%
Augmentation with Prostin	16	1.6%

Mode of Delivery		
Spontaneous Vaginal Deliveries	896	89.6%
Vacuum Extractions	90	9.0%
Caesarean Sections	14	1.4%

Onset of Labour		
Spontaneous Onset	952	95.2%
Inductions with Syntocinon	12	1.2%
Inductions with Prostin	33	3.3%
Inductions with Prostin + Syntocinon	3	0.3%

Perineum		
Intact Perineum	700	70.0%
Tears 1st degree	248	24.8%
Tears 2nd degree	29	2.9%
Tears 3rd degree	0	0.0%
Episiotomies	23	2.3%

Water Birth in Vienna: Facts, thoughts and philosophy of the Geburtshaus Nussdorf

Michael Adam is a gynaecologist and obstetrician, born in 1948 in a delivery room of the Women's University Clinic of Vienna. He was separated from his mother for three days. 'You don't need to see him, because you won't have milk until then,' were the reasons she was given. He considers his development of a very mother and child oriented approach to obstetrics to be due to this treatment. In 1986 he founded, together with a colleague and two midwives (today there are six midwives, six obstetricians and four paediatricians) the 'Geburtshaus Nussdorf' (the Birth House Nussdorf, an area on the outskirts of Vienna). More than 2000 babies have been born there, about ten per cent under water.

History

The Geburtshaus (Birth house) Nussdorf was founded as an initiative of four midwives and two obstetricians in 1986. Today we have six midwives and six obstetricians. In addition there are four paediatricians and several anaesthetists.

The six people had in common a dissatisfaction with obstetrics in their own environments; either in private or public hospitals, or in home birth. The doctors were dissatisfied with private hospitals because they saw the different interests between women and hospitals.

The easier the birth the less money for the hospital, therefore the more complicated births mean more money for the hospital (and the doctor).
Over all, an uncomplicated birth left us doctors redundant.

In the public hospitals the rigid structures were stronger than any individual who was interested in promoting change. Every change, to a more women oriented approach, was blocked with common arguments: 'we have no money' and 'we have always done it that way'.

Midwives had different reasons. Those coming from public backgrounds were tired of following obstetricians' orders, because they often thought they knew better (most of the time it was just to be more patient); and those coming from home births were more interested in co-operation with doctors, because they didn't want to transfer women to hospitals that often.

Thoughts and philosophy

Only two of the first four midwives who started working in Nussdorf were experienced in water birth. We doctors had only heard of, but had never seen, a water birth - even on a video. But the way the midwives reported on water during birth left us in no doubt of the fact that the birth will happen when it is supposed to happen. This was clear to us because we believe in the inner wisdom of the human body, and also in the inner wisdom of childbearing women.

From the very beginning, it was our goal to offer a supportive environment for labouring and delivering women. There is no alternative to what women think is good for them. So, if one thinks in a certain moment water is just the right thing, it is.

When it became widely known that water birth was an option in Nussdorf, more and more women chose Nussdorf for the birth of their baby. They knew water was the only place for them.

To those women who are adamant that the water is the only place for them, we suggest that it's better to be open for what will come, and not just to focus on the tub and nothing else. After nearly nine years' experience with water birth, we know that many of those who are sure that water is the only place for them, never give birth in the tub, because they get in far too early. But those who cannot even imagine using the tub, often change their minds towards the end of the first stage, and finally use the tub and then stay in to deliver the baby into the water, when they feel comfortable.

Giving birth in the water is a rather spectacular thing, but there is another part which is not spectacular at all but far more important: using the water as a relaxing pain relieving 'drug'. The majority of the women coming to our house are using the water for this purpose.

Summary

I want to give in short all the important details and results from our work in Nussdorf. First let me give you some information about the background in a little country like Austria, and how things have developed concerning water birth in the last ten years.

Austria is a little country in the heart of Europe. Until 1918 it was large and multicultural. More than 20 different people, speaking as many languages, lived within its borders. In the last century two of the main discoveries concerning childbirth were made by people who lived and worked in the Austro-Hungarian empire. One is unquestioned today, and many books are written about the faith of this man, though he was, during his lifetime, the obstetricians' enemy number one: Ignaz Semmelweis. He discovered the lethal effect of doctors coming from autopsies and then carrying out examinations on labouring women without any hygienic precautions. This fact caused the deaths of many women, usually only the poorest and often single women. Because of the shame of being pregnant and unmarried they were hidden, which meant giving birth at university clinics. Only there could doctors go from examining dead bodies to examining the living. Women who could afford it, of course, gave birth at home. Semmelweis's colleagues didn't appreciate it very much when he started accusing them of being responsible for the death of an uncounted number of young mothers. He died in a mad house under questionable circumstances.

The second discovery was made by Sigmund Freud, who, in his early years, 1897, stated 'Since the abnormal process of birth frequently produces no effect, one cannot exclude the possibility that, despite Little's anamnesis, diplegia might be of congenital origin. Difficult birth in itself in certain cases is merely a symptom of deeper effects that influenced the development of the fetus'.

What can one learn by the history of those men?

1.   One gets acknowledged in foreign countries rather than at home.
2.   As a minimum, he, she, or they, have to be dead. Because their achievements will not be recognized during their lifetime.

I do not consider us as important as the two eminent people I have mentioned before. But I do see us as a group of serious people, who are doing important work, without any acknowledgement from colleagues or health authorities, yet, on the other hand, we are known throughout the world.

In 1986, when we opened, we were considered irresponsible and crazy. But, as a matter of fact, the only thing we did was use midwives' experiences and follow the wishes of pregnant or birthing women. We questioned routine measures: routine enemas, routine episiotomies, routine electronic monitoring, routine lithotomy position for birth, and so on. We also introduced the possibility of water for giving birth in Vienna. We were lucky, and had two midwives in our staff who were experienced in water birth.

More interesting are probably different facts. I think our existence, alone, has changed Austrian, especially Viennese, obstetrics. People started to discuss things, and the hospitals came under pressure. Under this pressure things have change rapidly, either in one or the other direction.

The bad news first. In Upper Austria a gynaecologist, who had gathered lots of experience with water birth previously, and who wanted to practice water birth, found that when he became head of the obstetrical department, in a small Upper Austrian city, he was forbidden to do so by the Upper Austrian health authorities. No reason for this was given to him.

But let's switch to the good news. Routine enemas mostly don't exist any more. The rate of episiotomies went down enormously, in some hospitals it's now half as many as before. A consensus statement on continuous routine electronic fetal monitoring was worked out some years ago. It states the opinion of all Viennese obstetrical institutions on this issue and states that discontinuous monitoring is state of the art for monitoring fetal wellbeing during birth.

There is an increasing number of obstetricians who consider upright positions for giving birth as a valuable help to avoid vaginal operations and - that's why I am telling you all this - bath tubs are getting more and more routinely used to support dilatation. There is one big public hospital in Vienna which only recently invited Viennese gynaecologists to present first experiences with water birth. And, I understand, their experiences are excellent.

So, coming to the end, I want to summarize our point of view and experiences on water birth.

1.   Our experiences suggest that water birth is a useful technique and method for giving birth.
2.   It's safe if you follow certain rules.
3.   Finally, I want to emphasize what I have already mentioned at the beginning. If a woman comes and tells you she wants to give birth at your place we take the time to talk to her generally about birth. Though there are some women who know in every detail in advance what's good for them, the vast majority do not. Take time and speak about expectations and tell them that the art of childbearing is also the art of accepting things as they come. That can be water but it can also be something else.

My personal experience is that those women who say that water is especially for them usually don't give birth under water. This is because they are so concerned about the water they get into the tub much too early. After a while they get tired, want to do something else, and get out.

Those who can't imagine water birth at all are those who are more likely to give birth in the tub. As it's the other way round with these women they walk, lay down use whatever possibility we offer them, and finally often ask for the tub. Since the birth has usually progressed a long way by then, they often give birth under water. This is because when they get into the water they are nearly ready for the final thing - to let the new life change worlds: from inside the womb through the water into our world.

Some figures

We compared three groups of delivering women, looking mainly for complications in the mother and/or baby:

Group I	Women who never - neither during dilatation nor expulsion - used the tub
Group 2	Women who used water during dilatation only
Group 3	Women who gave birth under water

Table 14.1: Group 1, Group 2 and Group 3

Caesarean Section	Never in water	0.87%
	In water during dilatation	2.83%
Number of stitches after a tear		
None	Never in water	30.74%
	In water during dilatation	28.77%
	Birth under water	50.98%
1-3 stitches	Never in water	30.30%
	In water during dilatation	26.89%
	Birth under water	37.25%
More than 3 stitches	Never in water	38.96%
	In water during dilatation	44.34%
	Birth under water	11.76%
Over all stitches	Never in water	69.26%
	In water during dilatation	71.23%
	Birth under water	48.02%
3rd degree tear	Never in water	4.04%
	In water during dilatation	2.99%
	Birth under water	0.00%
Highest medication during dilatation		
None	Never in water	66.67%
	In water during dilatation	32.55%
	Birth under water	66.67%

Bach-Flowers and/or homeopathica	Never in water	21.21%
	In water during dilatation	37.26%
	Birth under water	25.49%
Spasmolytcs and/or Analgesics	Never in water	12.12%
	In water during dilatation	27.36%
	Birth under water	7.84%
Alkaloids	Never in water	0.00%
	In water during dilatation	2.83%
	Birth under water	0.00%
Spasmolytcs, Analgesics and/or Alkaloids	Never in water	12.12%
	In water during dilatation	30.19%
	Birth under water	7.84%
Allopathic drugs in the week after birth	Never in water	7.27%
	In water during dilatation	8.33%
	Birth under water	4.08%
Transferred newborns		
Within the first hour	Never in water	1.73%
	In water during dilatation	0.94%
	Birth under water	0.00%
From the birth centre	Never in water	1.30%
	In water during dilatation	1.89%
	Birth under water	0.00%
Over all transfers	Never in water	3.03%
	In water during dilatation	2.83%
	Birth under water	0.00%

Table 14.2: Water birth statistics May 1986 - February 1995

CHAPTER FIFTEEN

Water Birth in a Private Medical Hospital in France

> **Patrick Stora** after studying medicine at Bordeaux, was appointed intern in the French Caribbean and there encountered emergency medicine, not applicable to psycho-prophylaxis yet important for women who find themselves in emergency situations. So he went back to his region and noted the low priority accorded to prenatal assistance. He trained in Sophrology[1] and given the success he met, he was asked to practice birth in water. He observed the astonishing results of this method and the great demand from the public. Since then he has trained in perinatal Haptonomy using the same process for a better awareness among couples expecting a child.

Water as a symbol

I shall not develop the subject of the symbolism of water, other authors will have done that.

Significance of water in childbirth

I will pass briefly over the qualities of water and its benefits in giving birth:

- acceleration of the speed of dilation
- diminution of pain
- less medication: drugs and perfusion
- less frequency of use of forceps, ventouse, caesareans, episiotomies
- less haemorrhaging on delivery
- finally, excellent experience for women, of whom practically 100 per cent ask for this method of childbirth for their next pregnancy.

The water, the equipment

Here too, the importance of the water will have been developed, its temperature following strict rules (36–37.5 degrees), the type of pool having less importance. The question of infection has been resolved: there is no more than in classic childbirth. Finally, respect for contraindications in underwater delivery: prematurity, neonatal infection in particular.

On the other hand

I want to stress the results obtained by certain teams on the level of exit from the water of the primiparae at the moment of the 'expulsion': Why about 40–50 per cent of primips leave the water at that moment and this occurs, whatever type of pool is used and points of support have been installed.

I have drawn from this certain conclusions on the importance of the preparations for delivery being well organized: prenatal swimming and exercising in a swimming pool, yoga, sophrology and haptonomy, to mention but a few.

These preparations are intended to lead to an energetic and active delivery. Thus the woman plays an absorbing part in giving birth and will not 'suffer' it, which is perhaps the fundamental difference from a delivery under peridural analgesic, and it is also why the preparations are so important in such a delivery.

I will speak about preparations that I know best

Sophrology[1]

Preparing women to accept the idea of letting their child descend and accepting the idea of becoming a mother by techniques of relaxation and visualisation of the future: this is progressive Sophro-acceptance.

Haptonomy

It consists of a humane approach which, for Franz Veldman, its creator, recognizes affective contact which proves to be for the safety of the child and for its autonomy. Perhaps I will have the opportunity to develop this theme in the debate which follows. Haptonomy comes from the Greek, hapto: to touch and Nomos: science, so haptonomy is the science of touching, of affectivity. Haptonomy will give a woman and her companion the opportunity of guiding the child towards the outside world, and reassurance that it will itself find the way to its birth.

The mother and her child, after the reassuring attachment, will become aware of *the detachment of autonomy.*

These preparations will improve appreciably the efficiency of the pushing mechanism and subsequently the birth into the water. They do not affect the speed of dilation but the exiting of the child into the water by means of a better awareness of pushing, which 'liberates' the child.

But how will we be able to improve these results even more and also improve the women's experience?

---

1   The techniques of sophrology are included in the concept of hypnosis as is used in the English speaking countries.

The multi-disciplinary approach

I am convinced that childbirth in general cannot be approached in a narrow way, above all in the context of a medical establishment.

I will explain: in the more sensitive, more intimate birth at home, the physiology of childbirth is not as much disturbed by negative influences. Psychology and physical phenomena are closely linked in harmony.

To use an image, in a hospitalized confinement, the woman is fragmented. In a way she is a puzzle whose pieces are separated. Likening the woman to a puzzle is to respond in a remote fashion.

That cannot be satisfactory and only creates dystocia, difficulty in giving birth.

In the current context of hyper-specialization, the only means, in my opinion, of reconstituting this puzzle, of re-harmonizing the elements, psycho-affective, physiological and physical, of the woman is to work as a team.

Thus the sharing of the emotions, the dialogue with the couple shows that the vision must be wide, combining the participation of other practitioners, in particular those belonging to the so-called alternative medicines: homeopathy, acupuncture and Bach remedies, to only mention some, and this as part of the data on examination and the psycho-affective context.

We often have recourse to osteopathy which improves significantly the lombar-sciatic pains and corrects small pelvic anomalies, easing the descent of the baby at the delivery.

One or two consultations with a psychologist will be useful in some cases.

I will finish this presentation by coming back to more concrete matters about *indications* that are original and proper to aquatic childbirth:

- pre-eclamptic or eclamptic toxaemia
- narrow pelvises, it is common for babies of 3600g to be born to women with narrow pelvises
- anterior caesarean, and all the women in our series who had anterior caesareans, whatever the reason, have been able to give birth by natural means.

I expect from this conference and its participants some answers to the questions I ask myself.

There are obvious answers. Warm water allows:

- mental relaxation and a predominance of the electro-encephalographic alpha waves as is seen in relaxation techniques.
- a relaxation of the uterine muscle permitting a better labour using less energy, which is also why we observe fewer posterior (occipito-sacral) positions.

- a vasodilation for a better placentary perfusion.
- a better suppleness of the tissues, reducing the incidence of episiotomies and tears.

It can be pointed out here that the addition of salt to the bath water gives even better results.

But let us be vigilant, water has rules that must be respected. For my part, I rarely leave a woman in warm water for more than an hour and a half for a multipara and more than two hours for a primipara. This is the time usually necessary (and not more) to obtain a complete dilation when she re-enters the water at three or four centimetres.

Let the contributors reply to these questions on the basis of methodological and scientifically measurable and reproducible work, which in any case is the price we must pay in France for a recognition of aquatic birth, which it amply deserves.

Summary

The author summarizes in his presentation the contribution of water in childbirth and in particular the improvement of mechanical phenomena in labour, lessening medicalization.

He notes a large number of deliveries in water by primiparae for childbirth. For him, a prenatal preparation (sophrology and haptonomy) which is properly conducted makes women aware of letting their child descend, improving results. He thinks it necessary, in a medical environment, to have a multi-disciplinary approach to labour. He proposes specific indications for giving birth in water: toxemia, narrow pelvises and anterior caesareans. He hopes to have measurable responses explaining why giving birth in water gives so much satisfaction.

CHAPTER SIXTEEN

The Use of Warm Immersion in Labour at the Family Birthing Centre of Upland (California)

> **Michael Rosenthal** is a Board Certified obstetrician who opened the Family Birthing Centre of Upland in 1985 as an outgrowth of a private practice in a suburban Los Angeles community. Of the 3000 women admitted to the Centre almost 1000 of them gave birth in warm water. He has served as chairman of the obstetric department of the back-up community hospital. Since the Centre closed in 1994, Dr Rosenthal has been providing consultation to hospitals that are introducing warm water immersion. Dr Rosenthal lives in Claremont with his wife, Karen. One of their daughters attends Northwestern University. The other is enrolled at the University of Virginia Law School.

The Family Birthing Centre of Upland (FBC) opened its doors in January 1985 as an outgrowth of a large solo private obstetrical practice in a Southern California community located 35 miles east of downtown Los Angeles. It was the first centre in the United States to offer the option of warm water immersion (WWI) for pain relief in labour and birth. It soon gained a strong regional reputation as the only site at which this widely discussed option was available in this country.

There had been no prior hospital experience with this modality in this country. All of the other WWI experience had been associated with home birth and midwifery practice. It had finally appeared in the realm of standard obstetrical practice. It was introduced in an effort to move away from the tightening grasp of technological interventions in maternity care that were resulting in rising maternity care costs and in deteriorating birth outcome statistics, specifically increasing caesarean rates and increasing utilization of regional anaesthesia in labour.

There was no electronic fetal monitor in the Centre. Fetal heart tones were auscultated in accordance with the guidelines of the American College of Obstetricians and Gynaecologists. Women using the Centre recognized that midwifery, rather than obstetrics, was the standard of care.

The staff at the Centre consisted of two certified nurse midwives, six experienced labour and delivery nurses, four instructors in childbirth and lactation, and a support clerical and medical assistant staff of six. One obstetrician served as medical director providing care at the centre and at its back up hospital in the event of transfer.

Every two weeks orientation sessions, which were open to the general public, were held at the Centre. Slides and videotapes illustrating alternatives to hospital based birth complemented discussions of midwifery based care.

During the orientation discussions it was emphasized to potential clients that water birth is not a goal and WWI is not a 'method'. It is a treatment modality, much like medical analgesia or anaesthesia, that is one of several options available to women choosing to give birth at the Centre.

The FBC flourished because of its proximity to its back up hospital (150 yards), an appealing philosophy and style of care, and because of a growing reputation for good results, especially a low caesarean section rate and a high success rate of vaginal delivery among women who had previously had as many as three caesarean births.

Its clientele was largely middle to upper middle class, Anglo, educated and privately insured. Much of it was drawn from the more affluent communities of the region rather than the town of Upland itself. In the nine years of its operation there were noticeable shifts in the demographic characteristics of the surrounding community. It became increasingly Hispanic and blue collar. Based on interviews with the new arrivals, the FBC had no appeal. These were families who were seeking all the technology that they could get in the belief that they were entitled to the 'first class care' that their families, newly insured, could now afford.

After the first year of operation the FBC became a site for labour and birth available to women who had had a caesarean birth. Women were given the option of intensively monitored labour and proximity to the operating room in the hospital or the low tech approach offered to all 'normal' labouring women in the Centre. Almost all chose to be treated as though they were 'normal'. The result was a significant series of out-of-hospital Vaginal Birth After Caesarean (VBAC) deliveries.

In its peak years the FBC was a training site for nurse midwifery students in Southern California. It also provided hands-on experience and exposure to this new modality for groups of midwives from several European countries.

The Family Birthing Centre of Upland closed its doors February 25, 1994. This was primarily the result of the advent of managed health care schemes replacing traditional insurance. In this environment the key to survival is consolidation of health care providers into larger entities to enhance bargaining position. In large scale medicine the 'boutique' practices and personalized care offered by small entities, such as birthing centres, are excluded in favour of very large organizations whose focus is enhancing share-holder value.

A summary of the results

In nine years of operation there were 2970 women admitted to the FBC in labour. Of these 394 (13.2 per cent) were transferred to the back up hospital. There were 413 VBAC admissions; 13.9 per cent of the total. Primiparas represented 37.9 per cent (1126) and multiparas the remaining 62.1 per cent (1844). Roughly 60 per cent (1762) women laboured in water and about half of these (923) gave birth in the tub. Among all those admitted 324 (10.9 per cent) were eventually delivered by caesarean at the hospital.

Two hundred and fifty four of the primiparas (22.6 per cent) and 669 of the multiparas (36.3 per cent) gave birth in a tub.

Of the 2576 infants born at the centre 43 (1.7 per cent) were transferred to hospital. The greatest number (20) were sent to be observed for transient tachypnea of the newborn. One had meconium aspiration, three were diagnosed with lobar pneumonia, and one of these three had been waterborne. One had 'wet lung' two born in water had delayed recognition of torn cords at birth and became anaemic as a result. One of these required transfusion. This complication is probably unique to WWI for birth and it resulted in a policy of clamping the cord immediately whenever blood was seen in the water after a birth.

Major anomalies (4), testicular torsion (2), apnoeic episode (2), Apgar score less than 6 at 5 minutes (4), prematurity (3), and tachycardia (2) complete the list. One of the low Apgar infants was a tub birth.

There were 394 maternal transfers to hospital. Of the 279 transferred for failure to progress 264 eventually had a caesarean. Fifty-two received pitocin (oxytocin) augmentation and 21 of these were sections. Epidural anaesthesia was reason for transfer of 35 (1.2 per cent) women in labour and 18 of these had a section. The records do not clearly reflect why 13 were transferred. Passage of thick meconium (3), post partum haemorrhage (2), post partum eclampsia (1) and prolapsed cord (1) represent the remainder.

In our community approximately 80 per cent of all women admitted to hospital in labour receive analgesia during labour. At the FBC one narcotic, Stadol (butorphanol) was used exclusively and 515/2970 (17.3 per cent) received it. This relatively low rate was primarily attributed to lower maternal anxiety compared to the hospital, non-recumbent labour, enhanced maternal sense of control compared to the hospital, and the use of WWI.

Episiotomies were considered undesirable and to be avoided in all but 6 per cent of births. They were usually employed in conjunction with vacuum assistance observed in 133/2641 (5 per cent). Episiotomies following local anaesthesia were employed in five water births.

In 125 births there were 'complications' identified. Of 30 cases of tight nuchal cord 17 occurred in the tub. Of nine cases of shoulder dystocia only one was in the tub at the time. Two of the seven identified as having a malpresentation delivered in the water.

Overall there were 18 cases of retained placenta and seven of these were associated with water birth. Puerperal infection was identified in one woman who laboured briefly in water and one woman who never got into the tub. Blood loss in excess of 500 cubic centimetres was commented upon in 59 births. Two women experienced loss great enough to require transfusion.

Perineal injury rates were tallied with the following results. Among those who gave birth in water 27.8 per cent had no injury, 35.5 per cent had a first degree injury, 35.2 per cent had a second degree injury, 1.2 per cent had a third degree injury and only one had a fourth. Among those who did not labour in water 20.2 per cent had no injury, 28.2 per cent had a first degree, 49.5 per cent had a second degree, 3.7 per cent had a third and 1.6 per cent or 27 individuals had a fourth degree injury. This seeming excess of fourths was attributable to vacuum deliveries.

It was not felt that there were large enough numbers to make a meaningful statement about potential benefits of water birth in avoiding injury. However, there did not appear to be a trend to suggest benefit.

The Family Birthing Centre was the first in the country available to women who had previously had a caesarean. There was a total of 413 VBAC candidates admitted. Of the 341 who had only one section 67 (19.6 per cent) were sectioned again. Nine (15.5 per cent) of the 58 who had had two sections had another. Only one (7.7 per cent) of the thirteen who had previously had three sections required another. The one woman who had had four tried valiantly to avoid a fifth to no avail.

Overall, 81.9 per cent of all VBAC candidates had the vaginal delivery they had hoped for. This success rate is comparable to that achieved in other published series.

Conclusions

After observing many water labours and almost a thousand water births the question of its benefit is still not answered. To make any clear statement will probably require observation on a much larger scale and comparison to labour and birth in environments in which WWI is not available. A true prospective controlled study will probably never be possible, there are too many important factors such as anxiety levels and pain perception that do not lend themselves to easy quantification.

A major question posed by the positive comments of women who have had experience of water labour or birth is, 'Does warm water immersion in labour afford pain relief?' If it does, is it by influencing endorphin or catecholamine production? Does it work via altered neural transmission? To what degree do psychological factors mediate?

The fact that birth in water does not harm women or the infants born to them is clear, based on the observations at this Centre and in other larger series. It is tantalising to consider that water birth outcomes may actually be superior to those obtained in the high technology modern hospital environment. But, such a conclusion will wait for larger series and more observations in future studies.

CHAPTER SEVENTEEN

Labour and Birth in Water: An Obstetrician's Observations over a Decade

Faith Haddad is a Consultant Obstetrician and Gynaecologist. She graduated from Sheffield in 1967. Her MD was entitled Anxiety in Pregnancy. Faith was made a Fellow of the Royal College of Obstetricians and Gynaecologists in 1989, and she has been interested in 'Alternative' delivery positions since 1979 and actively involved in water births since 1987.

In late 1985 Yehudi Gordon and I decided to enter into partnership in private practice specializing in alternative delivery positions and the use of water during labour. At that time the Garden Hospital had a 'Jacuzzi' installed in the delivery room and occasionally a water birth occurred (unplanned). However, the pipe works of a Jacuzzi can not be completely sterilized and because of women's dissatisfaction at being asked to leave the Jacuzzi for delivery, we decided to replace this with a large specially designed pool. This occurred in 1987 and since that time women under our care have been free to deliver in water if medically appropriate.

In April 1992, the Garden Hospital closed the Birth Unit and Yehudi Gordon and I were fortunate in finding a new home for the Birth Unit at the Hospital of St. John and St. Elizabeth in St. John's Wood. The unit, on the third floor on St. Andrew's ward, has five rooms, four with double beds and two delivery rooms. Yehudi and I had worked with a group of midwives at the Garden Hospital and we moved as a team to John and Lizzies (as the hospital is more commonly called). Over the last three years the team spirit has been tested and strengthened and we are pleased to be here to present our work. The midwives have been responsible for collecting much of the data that I am presenting today and I would like to especially thank Mandy Kerr who has co-ordinated this. Lisa Beckles, the Birth Unit Secretary has also been invaluable. Suzie Kent and Karen Papier, our personal secretaries, have likewise played a major role in making this paper possible.

For this presentation, we chose to look at all the women who used water at some stage during their labour in 1993 and 1994. During this two year period 477 women delivered on the Birth Unit and 361 used water (76 per cent). There were a variety of reasons why some women did not use water, some women came in late in labour and there was insufficient time for them to use water, some had a complication contraindicating the use of water like intrapartum bleeding or pre-eclamptic toxaemia.

Firstly, I am going to tell you about what happened to the 365 women, in labour. Figure 17.1 shows the cervical dilatation at which women entered and left the pool. The majority, 63 per cent went into the pool before five centimetres dilation, which is earlier in labour than many advocates have suggested, and the majority, 60 per cent were advanced in labour or delivered before leaving the pool.

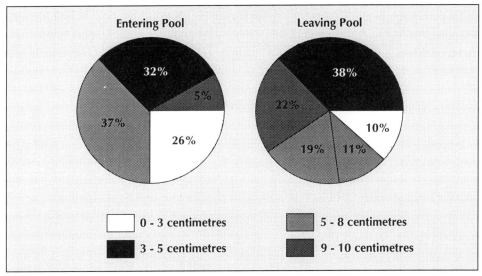

Fig. 17.1: Cervical dilatation

In Figure 17.2, if we look at the length of time women spent in the pool, we can see that 60 per cent spent more than one hour in the pool, and some used the pool intermittently.

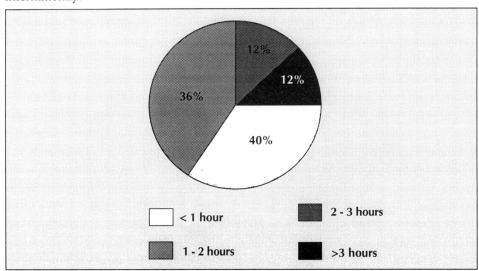

Fig. 17.2: Length of time in pool

The form of analgesia used is shown in Figure 17.3. For 68 per cent water was the only form needed (including massage, aromatherapy, homeopathy). Epidural analgesia was available at all times and 30 per cent of women requested this. Only three women had pethidine and a few used Entonox - some in the pool.

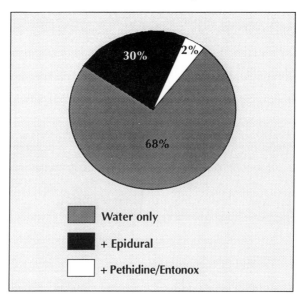

Fig. 17.3: Type of pain relief

In Figure 17.4, if we look at the mode of delivery, we can see that 88 per cent of women had a normal delivery and over a third of these were in the pool. Seven per cent had a forceps delivery and nearly five per cent required an emergency LSCS (Elective Caesarean Section did not use the pool and are therefore excluded from this analysis).

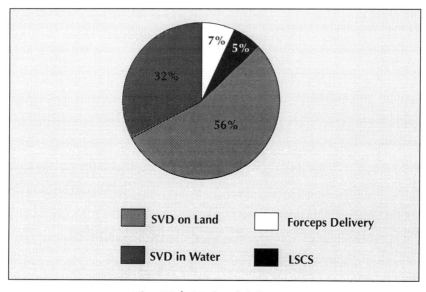

Fig. 17.4: Mode of delivery

The maternal position at birth is shown in Figure 17.5, and we can see that a variety of positions were chosen - some only possible in the pool, and some on land. The most common position in our unit for all deliveries was squatting, and in the pool, squatting, kneeling and floating were the most likely.

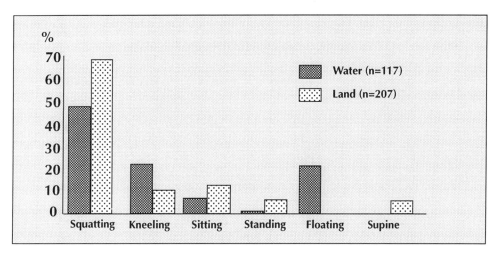

Fig. 17.5: Position at spontaneous birth

Figure 17.6 indicates the delivery of the placenta in relation to those women who delivered in the pool and 64 per cent remained in the pool for this: we found no complication as a result of this.

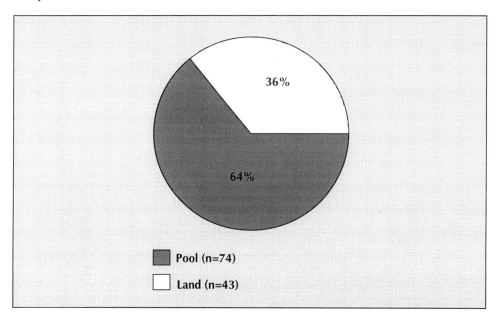

Fig. 17.6: Waterbirth - placental delivery

The outcome of the perineum is considered in Figure 17.7 in the pool. In the whole group, most women had an intact perineum or only a first degree tear. Those women who delivered in water were more likely to have an intact perineum or a first degree tear and less had a second degree tear, compared to the land births. Episiotomy, a fairly uncommon procedure, if not associated with a forceps delivery in our unit, was never carried out in the pool.

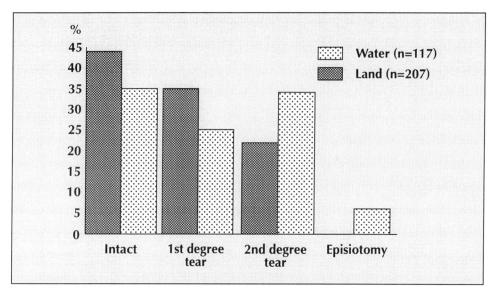

Fig. 17.7: Perineum in spontaneous birth

Neonatal outcome is a most important aspect of the assessment of water birth and Figure 17.8 shows the incidence of resuscitation in our unit in these 365 women. Babies born after more difficult labours, resulting in forceps deliveries and caesarean sections were most likely to require suction and oxygen; only one requiring intubation.

Neonatal Resuscitation				
	Water	Land SDV	Forceps and LSCS
Nil	110	193	31
Nasal O$_2$	7	13	9
Intubation	0	1	1
	117	207	41

Fig. 17.8: Neonatal resuscitation

Of the women who delivered in water, seven babies required some resuscitation in the first few minutes, but were, all but one, assessed as being fine at five minutes. The one baby, who was later transferred to SCBU (Fig.17.9) and intubed later, had an underdeveloped lungs and brain. This was a congenital abnormality, unfortunately incompatible with life, and the neonatal death was unrelated to the mode of delivery.

Transfer to SCBU	
Not transferred	358
Waterbirth	1
Spontaneous land birth	6
Forceps	1

Fig. 17.9: Transfer to SCBU

There were 12 babies reported to have neonatal infection of some description and only two of these were born in water.

This diagram shows the outcomes of a questionnaire which was sent by post to all of the 365 women and 190 women replied. The questionnaire asked women to rate their experience on a 9 point analogue score. The smaller number 1, being a lower response and the higher numbers 7, 8, and 9 being a greater response. We grouped the responses into three groups, i.e. 1-3 low, 4-6 medium and 7-9 high. In Figure 17.10 we show the responses to the four questions:

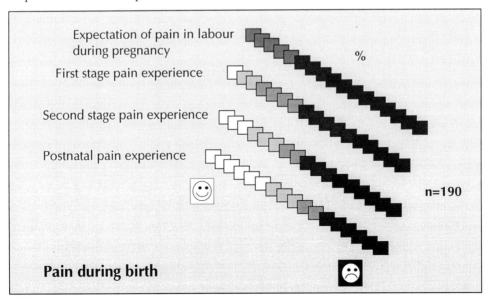

Fig. 17.10: Pain during birth

- How much pain in labour did you expect when you were pregnant?
- How much pain did you feel from the onset of labour up to the start of pushing the baby out?
- How much pain did you feel from the start of pushing your baby out up to the delivery of your baby?
- How much pain did you feel in the first 5 days after your baby was born?

You can see that women on the whole expected to feel more pain, than they actually describe feeling. Some women even describe the pain of the first stage of labour as being low, although the majority experienced high pain. The second stage of labour seems generally to have been perceived as less painful than the first stage, and there are factors here such as the use of epidural which may be involved. The postnatal perception of pain was much lower and this retrospective would be predicted and helps to validate the data.

We analysed the pain in the first stage of labour related to the use of analgesia (Fig.17. 11). For this analysis, low pain is 1-6 on the analogue scale and high pain is 7, 8 and 9.

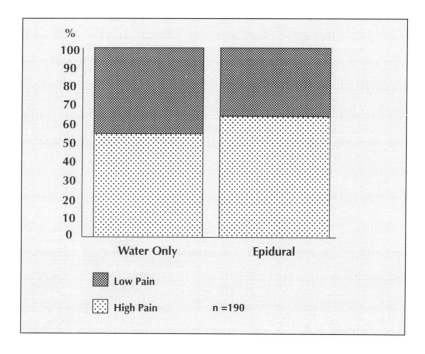

Fig. 17.11: Significant pain in the first stage

The women who used only water described their pain as being less than those who requested an epidural anaesthetic (Fig. 17.12). This was the case in the second stage of labour, where women who used an epidural perceived the pain to be much less.

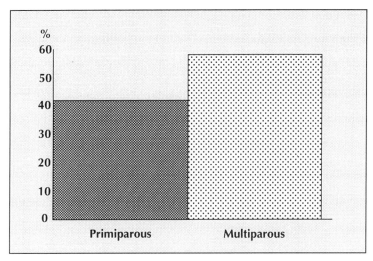

Fig. 17.12: Significant pain in the second stage

We looked at pain in the second stage of labour related to parity and found, surprisingly, that multips experienced more pain than primips. But again, this is related to the use of epidural analgesia as primips were more likely to have an epidural. (Experience of pain in the second stage of labour was not related to the type of delivery).

We asked women to rate the pain relief that they got from using the pool and Figure 17.13 shows their responses in relation to parity. Low pain is 1-3, medium 4-6 and high 7-9. The pain relief was assessed as being high (55 per cent) for multips and high for 40 per cent of primips. Each square represents five per cent of the pool group.

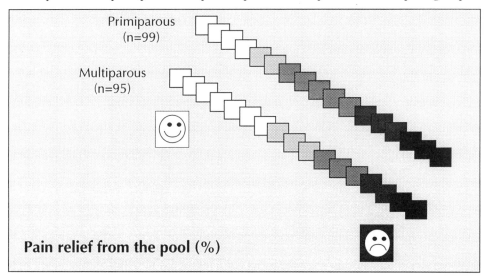

Fig. 17.13: Pain relief from the pool

Also a greater number of primips found the pool to be of low benefit in the relief of pain than the multips.

In Figure 17.14 we have looked at the women who rate the relief of pain in the pool as being high i.e. 7, 8 & 9 in relation to the use of water and epidural analgesia. Not surprisingly the number of women who found water to give high pain relief was greater in those who used water only.

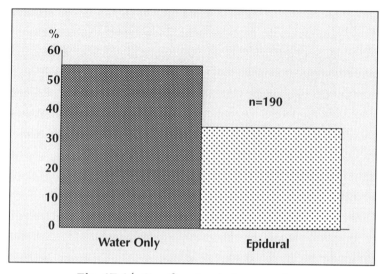

Fig. 17.14: Significant pain in second stage

The women who found high pain relief in the pool were more likely to stay in the pool for delivery (Fig. 17.15), and much less likely to have a forceps delivery or caesarean section.

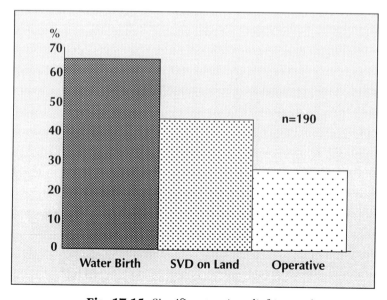

Fig. 17.15: Significant pain relief in pool

Also, the women who found high pain relief in the pool were more likely to have a favourable outcome as far as the perineum was concerned (Fig. 17.16). This is, of course, related to the higher water birth rate in this group and low episiotomy rate in women who found effective pain relief in the pool.

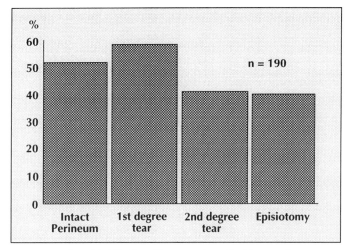

Fig. 17.16: Significant pain relief in pool

When we looked at women who had a lot of postnatal pain (7, 8 & 9 on the analogue score) this related to what had happened to the perineum at delivery. Those with an intact perineum (18 per cent) or first degree tear (12 per cent) experienced less pain, than those with second degree tears (15 per cent) and even less than those with an episiotomy (38 per cent). Why women with a first degree tear complained less than those with an intact perineum is a mystery.

Women were asked to grade the attention they received from the midwives during labour (Fig. 17.17) and the vast majority rated it as high (7, 8 & 9).

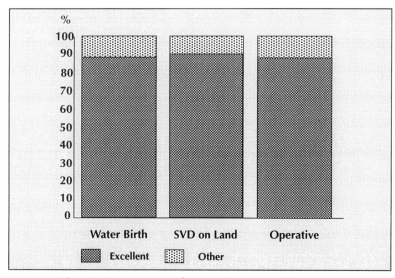

Fig. 17.17: Attention from midwives in labour

The lighter area is all those who rate it as less than 7. The attention from the midwives did not vary significantly according to parity, type of analgesia or type of delivery. Therefore, if we consider that the midwives gave equally good attention to all the women, who can exclude the role of the doula as a variable outcome of labour?

In view of the publicity in recent years about the safety issues relating to water birth, we wondered how much this may affect women. Therefore, we asked women to rate the influence of media reports. The responses are shown here (Fig. 17.18). The groups in light shades are low influence (1-3) and the dark shades are medium (4-6) and high (7-9). Each square again represents five per cent of the group.

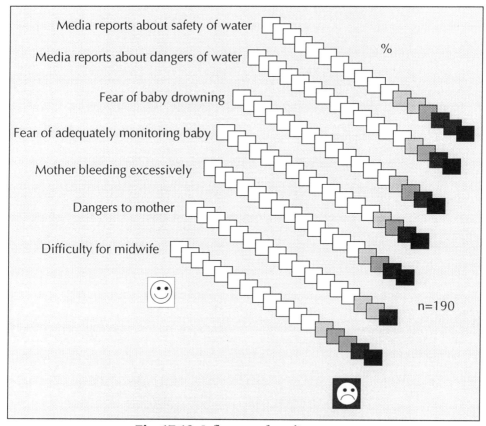

Fig. 17.18: Influence of media reports

- How do you feel media reports about the safety of water birth influenced your attitudes to the use of water?
- Were you influenced by media reports about the dangers of water birth?
- How concerned were you that your baby might drown in the pool?
- How concerned were you that your baby would be adequately monitored in the pool?
- How concerned were you about bleeding excessively in the pool?
- How concerned were you about danger to yourself using the pool?
- How concerned were you that using the pool could make it difficult for the midwife to attend to you or your baby?

Figure 17.18 shows that the majority of women, 75 per cent, were little influenced by media reports. Of course, this is a retrospective questionnaire and is answered by women who choose to come to a private unit which specializes in water birth.

In Figure 17.19 we have looked at those women who had high concern about media reports about the safety of water birth (7-9) compared to low concern (1-6) in relation to the mode of delivery. Women with high concern seemed equally likely to have a water birth or a spontaneous vaginal delivery on land, but less likely to have an operative delivery. This is interesting, but probably not significant statistically as the numbers are small in the operative delivery group (11 per cent).

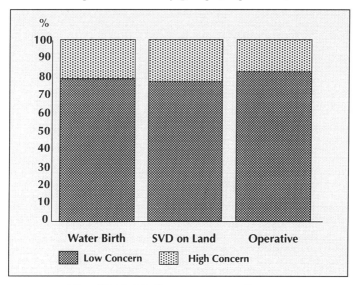

Fig. 17.19: Media reports on safety

Lastly, we asked women to rate their overall birth experience, and again, excellent is 78 per cent with 1-6 being the rest (Fig. 17.20).

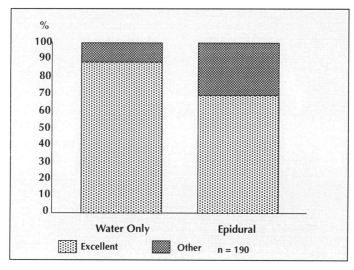

Fig. 17.20: Mother's rating of the birth experience

Overall the birth experience was considered to be very good by the majority, but those who used only water were more likely to be satisfied than those who chose to have an epidural. Similarly perceived good birth experience was greater in those who had a water birth, compared to those who had a normal delivery on land (Fig. 17.21). The women who had a forceps delivery or caesarean section were less likely to perceive their birth experience positively, but nevertheless over 50 per cent of them did.

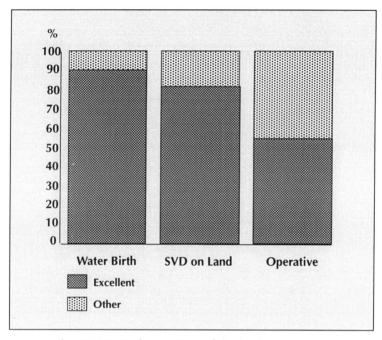

Fig. 17.21: Mothers rating of the birth experience

Women's perceptions about water birth have not received much attention from researchers as yet and this pilot study might stimulate others to look in more depth in this area. Another aspect which has never been looked at is to question the birth attendants about their views.

PART SEVEN

Water Birth Internationally

CHAPTER EIGHTEEN

Water Birth in Australia

Athena J. Vassie is a registered nurse/midwife. Her general training took place at King's College London and her midwifery in Plymouth. She has been working as a midwife since 1984. In 1986 she moved to Sydney, Australia, and worked for five and a half years in a midwifery run Birth Centre attached to a women's public hospital in the city. This was open to both private and non-fee paying public clients, regardless of where they lived (or economic status). The Centre catches over 400 babies a year. Athena has now retired to look after her own water baby.

I have been invited to share my experience of water birth and to report on what is happening in Australia at this time. I have worked in an active birth centre for the last five years. It is a midwifery run unit and has over 80 per cent public clients, allowing us more freedom to facilitate their needs. I am a member of a team that has attended over 150 water births in the last few years. Our average length of labour for a primip is nine and a half hours and multip six hours. We have had two babies born with an Apgar score below seven at one minute and two other babies were admitted to neonatal care febrile and tachypnoeic. Six women have had post partum haemorrhages in the bath, one of 2000mls. All recovered well. Statistics show less perineal trauma with water birth. We have had no third degree tears or episiotomies.

In Australia, a large number of babies are well over 4kgs at birth. We have had one episode of shoulder dystocia. The baby weighed 4280gms, with Apgar scores of seven and nine. Eighteen per cent of our water babies weigh over 4kgs. Less than six per cent weigh under 3kgs. Our largest water baby to date weighed 4675gms; it was the mother's first.

Other water births of note were: One mother who chose to labour and birth in the bath following a known intra-uterine death and induction of labour, plus undiagnosed twins which were born 20 minutes apart with no problems.

Australian Telecom yellow pages was used to access information on hospitals providing maternity services. I sent out 229 questionnaires to hospitals all over the country. It can take four hours to fly either north-south or east-west. Obviously, some hospitals were going to be doing minimal obstetrics. I also sent out 100 questionnaires to subscribers of the Australian Society for Independent Midwives (ASIM). Although not all of these would practice independently, response rates were very good, 78 per cent from hospitals and 77 per cent from the independents.

Geographically, we are at a disadvantage in Australia, due to large distances to travel to receive care, and, in remote areas, reduced facilities. Australia is almost the same size as the United States, but with a population of only 17 million in comparison to the States 260 million.

In Australia, small rural hospitals may have less than 20 births per annum, and are staffed by GPs and midwives for low risk pregnancies. A supra regional hospital covers all levels of obstetric risk and provides neonatal intensive care. They are referral centres for all levels of obstetric/neonatal country transfers and they have more than 3,500 deliveries per annum. They are staffed by specialist obstetricians and midwives.

Water births seem to be a very emotive subject in Australia. Most midwives, doctors and consumers think it is best avoided at all costs; a view based on ignorance rather than scientific knowledge.

I was amused, but not surprised, to read some of the comments when asked 'Do you have any unspoken rules or conditions to not birth in water that may not be official hospital policy?'

Some were:

- poor water supply,
- women not educated for water birth antenatally,
- no room in bath,
- bath removed for hygienic reasons,
- told when opening birth centre that there were to be no water births as hospital insurance not adequate, not practised and not likely to be practised at this facility,
- doctors state it will not take place,
- feel it is simply a matter of time,
- interested; there is a demand but not talked about in case they ban it.

Interestingly, a number of midwives who returned the questionnaire say the reason water births do not take place is either:

- no client request,
- management or doctors, yet few midwives would feel happy or competent to participate in water birth.

A rural hospital stated it was not appropriate due to their remote location. They obviously consider water birth a dangerous practice.

It would also seem that of those hospitals with a bath available, for the most part less than one third of women used it in labour on a regular basis. The best result for bath usage, so far, is in Tasmania, where it rose as high as 95 per cent in one hospital, although it is used most frequently in NSW, Victoria and Tasmania.

One has to wonder if midwives ever think to suggest to a labouring woman that baths may help with pain relief. That they could fail to be aware of the benefits to both mother and baby I find hard to believe, as the overwhelming response when asked if midwives felt drug usage was less with using a bath for pain relief was, and is, yes. It would seem to me that if this is what midwives believe, baths as a tool for coping with pain should be promoted; to give babies a healthier start to life and to be looked after by an alert, drug free mother.

As for hospitals even thinking ahead to the possibility of water births, very few have encompassed the idea. However, one hospital sticks out by having a policy on water birth though at this time they do not have a bath!

As for doctors being willing to participate in water birth, for the whole country 16 have been estimated by the midwives to be possible candidates. This is only doctors practising in a hospital setting, not the community.

Now, to look at actual water births in Australia, and yes we have had a few, some hospitals more than others.

New South Wales (NSW)

Most hospitals participating in water birth in NSW say they are 'unplanned', probably to protect themselves. In these hospitals, bath usage varies from between 50-95 per cent. Midwives at these hospitals say they are mostly uncomfortable with the idea of water birth, although one birth centre has 100 per cent support from its midwives. It would seem the more water births seen, the more likely a midwife is to participate. Out of six hospitals who participate in water birth in NSW only three have a policy in place. Two hospitals have doctors likely to be present at a private client's water birth, they do not appear comfortable with this event. Delivery rates vary between 120-1000 per annum in centres where there is a bath available. In hospitals where there is a labour ward and a birth centre, all water births take place in the birth centres. All seem to have occurred in the 1990s with the exception of one hospital, with an unknown number of water births from 1985, with problems which were not stated. One hospital has a water birth rate of approximately 18 per cent of all deliveries.

Tasmania

The smallest state in Australia, with six hospitals targeted and very limited choices available to women, seems to be a progressive advocate for women and their right to self determined care. Two hospitals have participated in water birth since the 1990s. One hospital has support from their obstetricians for water birth, and admit to planned water birth for both public and private clients. 60-95 per cent of labouring women use the bath. In those hospitals where water birth is practised, the numbers of midwives who were comfortable with the idea of water birth varied from only one per cent in one hospital to 80 per cent. One hospital only has a policy in place. Delivery rates vary between 800-1700 per annum in these hospitals.

Victoria

Of the hospitals in Victoria which are known to participate in water birth, most would appear to be unplanned. The first water birth was as early as 1978, but none has since occurred at this hospital, so it seems safe to assume they are not in favour. However, most water births have occurred in the 1990s. Bath usage by labouring women varies between 3-90 per cent in these hospitals. Few midwives are comfortable with the idea. Two hospitals have a policy on water birth. Labour wards and birth centres vary in size from one to six beds. No maternal or fetal problems have been noted. There is one private free standing birth centre which has been participating in water births since 1983. They noted lower Apgar scores if the water was too hot. Delivery rates vary between 40-2000 per annum in these hospitals.

South Australia

Only one hospital has admitted to water births so far, both 'unplanned'. The bath is in the birth centre and is used by 70 per cent of those clients. Labour ward clients may only access the bath when the birth centre is not using it, therefore only 10 per cent get this option. The hospital does not allow water births but does have an emergency procedure should one take place (not stated). Few midwives are comfortable with the idea of water birth, but believe two doctors would support it if the hospital had a policy supporting water birth.

Western Australia

Western Australia has only had one water birth so far in a hospital (I have since found out, informally, that others have taken place, how many I do not know). 50 per cent of labouring women use the bath. 75 per cent of midwives at this hospital would be happy to participate in water birth. However, medical officers do not encourage use of the bath. They also have no policy on water birth.

As to independent midwife practice, this seems to be where the majority of water births are happening. Midwives around the country use the bath for pain relief extensively; between 35-90 per cent for the most part. Clients booked per year can vary from as few as one up to 70 with an average of 20-30. Most midwives work alone.

Only four independent midwives around Australia felt uncomfortable participating in water birth. Three of these were from New South Wales, a state with many independent midwives, though I only accessed 24 of them. NSW is also more than six times the size of England.

The other midwife uncomfortable with water birth lives in Western Australia, a state covering one third of Australia, and over nineteen times the size of England. I had replies from six independent midwives in Western Australia but, again, I am unsure just how many practice independently. The size of the state obviously adds constraints to this practice.

Reasons given for advice against water birth were fetal distress, breech, thick meconium, maternal skin infections, suspected shoulder dystocia and midwife anxiety.

Water births have been recorded from as early as 1970 in Western Australia and 1979 in Victoria, with the majority taking place in the 1990s. There have been minimal problems with only one reported episode of an asphyxiated baby, which survived. This was in New South Wales. To date, and to my knowledge, the number of water births which have taken place with independent midwives are:

- Western Australia   112
- New Territories   20
- New South Wales   203
- ACT (Australian Capital Territory)   1
- Victoria   265
- South Australia - Tasmania   13
- Queensland   124

The percentage of births as water births with independent midwives varies from 1-65 per cent. There are a few lay midwives in Australia, these are individuals who have no formal hospital or university based training. These lay midwives are now illegal in some states.

Summary

Obviously these figures apply only to my survey, as I could only access midwives practising independently who subscribe to ASIM. There are probably many more whose water births will go uncounted. The hospital figures are probably not complete, as I had to make a decision as to which hospitals to send my questionnaire to. However, I do feel I probably accessed the vast majority of relevant hospitals.

I would like to finish with a reflection on the difficulties faced by Australian midwives, trying to facilitate the needs of their clients, in a country with a population of only 17 million but with a land mass 59 times the size of England. Can we blame midwives for feeling uncomfortable with the idea of water birth when they have little hope of ever being present at such an event, and where there has been little research and virtually no education on the subject? How, therefore, are they to gain their own skills and confidence and to use those skills to educate others?

CHAPTER NINETEEN

Water Birth in Italy

Piera Maghella has been an Active Birth Educator since 1980 and founded an Active Birth Centre in Modena (MIPA). It offers birth preparation courses for women and couples from the beginning of pregnancy and support in the postnatal period with an SOS telephone system. She conducts seminars and workshops for professionals in private settings and in hospitals (December 94 in 69 Italian Public Hospital) She is Director of a Newsletter *Nascita Attiva* and produces material and aids for antenatal education. She has written three books. *Preprazions al parto attivo*, a manual for consumers, *Come organizzare e condurre un corso*, a manual for professionals on how to lead a group and *Stretching per la gravidanza*. Piera attends many births as a 'Doula' and she has three children.

Italy is a strange country! Full of conflicts! Generally speaking one could summarize birth in Italy by saying that:

'Even though, for religious and cultural reasons the family is very important, Italy is the country that has the lowest birth rate in the world! People have less children for socio-economical reasons, but we should also consider the traumatic experience women have during a very medicalized birth and their isolation in the postnatal period.

The Italian situation is very medicalized. For example: during pregnancy women receive at least three ultrasounds routinely - in many cases every month; women are given an internal every time they go to the doctor; for birth, 99.9 per cent of women go to hospitals and there they are monitored continuously, even when walking; too many women are still made to lie on their back to give birth and have a routine episiotomy; babies are medicalized, as they are kept in the nursery; breastfeeding is not supported and bottles are given out far too easily.

It is so medicalized that we have the highest rate of caesarean sections in Europe, and we are the second in the world after Brazil. Nationally, the rate is 25 per cent, but with very different statistics for state hospitals and private ones. An example: the Region of Lazio, where Rome is, has more than 30 per cent caesarean sections in public hospitals and 42 per cent for the private ones.

Italy has the highest number of doctors per inhabitant, and too many obstetricians. In every hospital, very often, the number of doctors present in the labour ward is the same, or more, than the number of midwives. Many doctors, even professors at teaching hospitals, are not very up to date with scientific trials, and personal experience is put forward as the most relevant and valid. So many doctors have many things to do. Many caesarean sections and lots of anxiety during birth.

The midwife has a very low profile, and her role is very often that of an auxiliary for the obstetrician. In general, midwives are not very political therefore they exert little pressure. Generally speaking, women see the midwife only when they enter the hospital during labour. As the doctor is the person the woman sees during pregnancy, as a consequence she hopes to see him/her there at the birth. A few groups of midwives that can be considered 'radical' see women during the entire pregnancy, labour, and the difficult transitional period after the birth.

There are very few home births, and recently none, assisted by the midwives in the public Health Service. They are all privately assisted. In two regions the Councils pay part of the cost. The issue of home birth is very hot, and usually stimulates lots of discussions and very irrational reactions.

We have 83 consumer groups connected to childbirth, but only a few of them are strong consumer groups. They are formed mainly by small numbers of good midwives who are quite isolated, and the idea of networking is not very strong.

To sum up, you can say that most of the land in Italy is surrounded by water - the sea, yet we have very few water births and those that occur take place in hospitals far away from the sea!'

Although this overview seems very pessimistic, I should say that a few things have been changing since the beginning of the 1980s. In many areas there are now more groups. In hospitals partners are allowed to stay all the time, women can walk about during labour and even use comfortable positions, and babies are given to the mother immediately after birth, but not for long.

At the beginning of the 1990s we had a few public hospitals (about 20 and mainly in the North), quite small ones (around 400/600 births a year). Thanks to a few professionals (midwives or doctors), and helped by the requests of women and couples, women started to be treated in a more human way and with a more scientific approach. These hospitals set up 'family rooms' which can be described as home-like birthing rooms with a lower and larger bed, cushions, with the Dutch birth stools, closed doors, low lights. A few of these 'Humanized Hospitals' doubled their number of births as women travelled to have a freer and more active labour, and they have been used as a model for more hospitals - but everything is very slow.

After a few successful years, these hospitals installed birthing pools and from 1990/91 we started to have water births. Since then, we have collected data on approximately 1000 births in water.

Regarding water birth, many hospitals are now allowing women to soak in water during some of the final hours of labour, and some have big, comfortable, appropriate pools. More hospitals have normal homelike baths and usually at night (when doctors sleep) women can get the benefit of the warm water.

Geographically speaking, hospitals which offer the possibility of water births are located as follows:

In the North of Italy, towards France, there are three hospitals:

In the province of Turin with Chieri (52 per cent labour in water, 30 per cent give birth in water with approximately 500 births a year), Chieri is very similar and Moncalieri is a much bigger hospital (1600 births a year) with 30 births in water in 1994. Very recently in Torino, the biggest teaching hospital with 4,000 births a year, women are allowed to soak in water.

Near Milan we have a private hospital in Varese with a few births in water and in Milan we have the unique Home Birth Centre (private, but very accessible), the Casa della madre e Fanciullo has very few water births, but many labours in water.

Towards Lake Garda we have Gavardo, a hospital with a few births in water. In the Region of Bologna we have two hospitals with important figures: Correggio is very near my town and has approximately 100 births a year, and Forli which, since 1989, has had approximately eight per cent of its births in water (with 900 births a year).

In Tuscany, where Florence is, we have Poggibionsi - one of our historical and model hospitals in the process of humanisation of birth with approximately 100 births since 1991, the year they installed the pool, and Castiglion Fiorentino has had 31 births.

In Rome, a very timid adventure is taking place in a big hospital. The actual assistance is very timid and with a huge internal conflict about safety, but the publicity has been very big!

Then, going South, we have a day hospital in Lecce, at the very bottom of the heel of Italy, where there has been a few water birth experiences and in Calabria in the beautiful mountains, 16 per cent of births have been in water.

And of course, in some home births, water is used with familiar equipment both in labour and in the second stage.

Thanks to books, the media, women travelling to different hospitals, seminars and conferences, we hear that more hospitals are offering the possibility of using water and some of these state hospitals are university hospitals. We hope that these will contribute and offer a different approach so that it will become acceptable to the medical establishment.

The effects of water, according to the hospitals that are offering it, are as follows: the percentage of caesarean sections has lowered, in one case from 23 per cent to 17 per cent in one year; the use of water is preferred for primigravida, those expecting their first child; there is analgesic effect; the length of the first stage is shorter; there are more intact perineum, very few tears; less procedures; longer second stage; babies slightly more blue at birth but their Apgar scores are fine.

Women's experiences are very encouraging and the most common expression is, 'It was wonderful!'. They feel the immediate comfortable effect of warm water, feeling less pain, freer in their movements, feeling contained and more in symbiosis with their baby, somehow less emotionally inhibited. They feel that the water and the pool is a positive barrier against medical procedures, internal examinations and people in general. Women feel more in control. Some women have now bought big, plastic, round, cheap containers (the ones used for the grapes when producing wine) for their home birth, and some women have even offered, as a present, a birth pool to the hospital in which they choose to give birth!

Partners, in many water births, felt excluded as they could not enter the water themselves or their women would not allow them, but they are still fascinated by the power of water.

To conclude, in the Italian situation water birth could be a very good way to introduce active birth by which we mean a self-searching and self-management process of giving birth for women. Women could protect themselves and at the same time feel contained by the water. I also feel that for many doctors, physiological births, natural births or active births are difficult to accept as they need to wait, to put their hands in their pockets, to believe in women's profound resources, and to get involved emotionally by the experience and not to use machines and technology, the left brain!

But water birth, although it is very feminine, sensual and mothering in its essence, could keep them men quiet! With the water, the pool, the installation of the plumbing system, the thermostat, the pipes, the project, the money involved. Maybe these aspects would enable them to satisfy their desires for technology and money spending projects.

Professionals don't like to get wet, or to use long gloves, therefore women are saved by being subject to less procedures.

But in all this there is the risk that water and the pool in these circumstances becomes more important than the birth and the experience itself for the women and the professionals! There is the risk, in these first births in water, that instead of it being a more intimate, protective and private experience that the use of water being so new and topical may attract too many nervous people: more doctors, neonatologists, anaesthetists.

Water birth should be one of the many elements and external resources that women can use if they want to have a nice, deep, intense and global experience.

CHAPTER TWENTY

Water Birth in Denmark

Anne Uller is a mother of three children and since 1993 has been Head of Midwifery, Fåborg Maternity Unit. She began to work with water births in 1993 and started an official programme of water birth. She has worked to inform the public about the outcomes of water births, and the number of water births in the hospital has increased to almost 36 per cent during the past year. She has purchased a third water tub for use at home births to support those who choose not to go to hospital. Freedom of choice when giving birth is of greatest importance to her, and is the main reason for her involvement in water births.

I am very pleased to have been invited to this conference, as it gives me a unique opportunity to share our experiences of the use of water during labour and birth with the rest of the world. We have eight midwives in Fåborg, all of them are attending this conference.

In my presentation I will tell you about:

1. The experience with water birth in Denmark in general.
2. About water births in Fåborg in particular.

Water births in Denmark

The use of water during labour has been practised in Denmark for many years. During the past five years the use of water during birth has become increasingly popular, and interest among women giving birth, as well as professionals, is growing.

In the beginning, only a few private practising midwives attended water births at home, they shared their experiences with the rest of us, and did a good job of 'promoting' water births in Denmark.

With the help of several parents, and a Danish Trust, similar to the National Childbirth Trust (a childbirth education organization in the UK), their efforts have resulted in bringing water births into several hospitals, as more and more women and midwives have learned about the advantages of using water during birth.

The following table shows that there are five large obstetric and five small maternity units with an official programme of water births (11 of the 52 Danish birth units).

Including the estimated 50 home births from all over the country, there has been a total of approximately 500 water births in Denmark in 1994, most of them taking place in small maternity units:

Obstetric units			
Glostrup:	10/3000 deliveries/year	0.03%	
Gentofte:	22/2500 deliveries/year	1.00%	
Roskilde:	75/2600 deliveries/year	3.00%	
Odense:	10/3700 deliveries/year	0.25%	(start Nov. 1994)
Svendborg:	35/1100 deliveries/year	3.50%	
Total:	152	34%	
Small maternity units (units in local hospitals with no obstetricians attached, mainly run by midwives, with a backup of general surgical consultants)			
Hobro:	45/425 deliveries/year	10.90%	
Grindsted:	27/650 deliveries/year	4.00%	
Samsø:	2/36 deliveries/year	5.00%	(small island)
Ringkøbing:	15/250 deliveries/year	4.00%	
Nyborg:	35/300 deliveries/year	11.00%	
Fåborg:	169/475 deliveries/year	35.00%	
Total:	293	56%	
Home births			
In water:	app.50	10%	

Table 20.1: Obstetric units and small maternity units

A few other places have also had some water births, but they have done so without official approval. They are all working at establishing an official programme in the near future, and I am sure they will succeed.

The main obstacles in the places wanting to start water births are doctors. There is a widespread scepticism among obstetricians, paediatricians, and microbiologists. Their main concern seems to be infection, aspiration and laceration, mainly because there is no substantial scientific research on the subject. But there are also midwives who object to attending water births. The main arguments are the 'difficult' working positions, the idea of water births being unhygienic, the fear of infection in times of HIV, the issue of safety for mother and child, and, perhaps, the general fear of trying something new and unknown.

When asked, the National Health Board of Denmark had no objection to water births. There have been no reports of neonatal deaths due to the use of water, but the Health Board is not yet willing - or ready - to give general guidelines for water births to every birth unit.

The only problem mentioned when talking to the different birth units is that there has been incidents where the umbilical cord unexpectedly snapped. In Gentofte they have had two, in Roskilde, three, and in Fåborg we have had two in 234 water births. They caused no serious problems for the baby, and we do not know how often this happens in bedside births. But in order to prevent any problems of this kind, we are cautious not to put too much water in the tub. If the water is too deep and the cord is very short, the baby cannot come to the surface. Until you find out about this you might have pulled too much on the cord!

In Roskilde, the first obstetric unit with an official water birth programme (since 1st January, 1993) a group of midwives, doctors and microbiologists are just about to start a project investigating infection. They hope to get results from 100 water births and a similar control group.

There is still no thorough registration of all water births in Denmark, but it could be done quite easily through the existing national birth register.

Although giving birth in water is still not very common, the use of warm water during labour is very well established. Almost all of the Danish birth units have one or several water tubs, and made frequent use of it for pain relief and relaxation. It is estimated that more than 50 per cent of all Danish women are in the water for a short or longer period when in labour.

Water births in Fåborg

The maternity unit in Fåborg is a small maternity unit, within the local public hospital, with approximately 500 deliveries a year.

We have eight midwives and a number of general surgical doctors, but no obstetricians are attached. Only low risk women are admitted to our unit, but we are able to handle the most common complications such as caesarean section and ventouse. We don't use forceps, we have no equipment for electronic fetal monitoring, fortunately. We don't use epidurals for vaginal deliveries, but we do prefer to do spinals for all caesarean sections (including emergencies).

Water births began in September 1993, and since then there have been a total of 234 water births. In 1994 we had 169, which were 35 - 58 per cent of all deliveries. 71 - 58 per cent of all women were in the water tub during labour, and 49 - 56 per cent of these actually gave birth in the water.

According to our *guidelines for water birth* any healthy woman at term expecting a healthy baby in a vertex presentation with an uncomplicated labour, having had no pethidine, can deliver in the water if she wants (see guidelines p.128).

The major effect of frequent use of water has been to decrease the use of medication and the need to intervene in the process of birth. Table 20.2 below shows the change:

Births in Fåborg				
	1993		**1994**	
Births in Total	440	100.00%	475	100.00%
Labial/vaginal/perineal trauma	209	47.50%	277	58.32%
Episiotomy	78	17.73%	43	9.05%
3rd degree tear	10	2.27%	3	0.63%
Syntocinon infusion	86	9.55%	64	13.47%
Entonox	94	21.36%	40	8.42%
Pethidine	24	5.45%	12	2.53%
Pudendal block	29	6.59%	20	4.21%
Local anaesthetic	40	9.09%	25	5.26%
Water tub	252	57.27%	340	71.58%
Water birth	14	3.18%	169	35.58%
Ventouse	34	7.73%	25	5.26%
Planned caesarean section	16	3.64%	14	2.95%
Emergency caesarean section	38	8.64%	31	6.53%
Total caesarean section	54	12.27%	45	9.47%
Home births	15	3.41%	12	2.53%

Table 20.2: Births in Fåborg

Most remarkable is the decrease in the number of episiotomies and third degree tears, the decrease in syntocinon infusion and the use of Entonox and pethidine. We seek to diminish the use of pethidine even more.

In order to watch water births closely we have made detailed registration of them all (243 water births).

In our experience water birth has been proven to be good and safe for both mother and child. 98 - 72 per cent of the water born children have had an Apgar score of 7-10 after one minute, and 99 - 57 per cent have had a score of 10 after five minutes. Only one baby had a low Apgar score of 5/1 -7/5 due to meconium aspiration. He was transferred to the nearest special care unit, where he recovered very fast.

We have had no reports of infection due to the use of water, no increase in the number of perineal tears - they are mainly small first degree tears - and no increase in the numbers of post partum haemorrhage.

The women have all been very pleased with their water births and the possibility of being in the water during labour. To us, the most important issue is actually the women's freedom of choice when in labour, and not whether she is having a water birth. No special preparation is required during pregnancy, but we talk about the possibility of being in water when we are asked, and we have made an information folder for anyone interested.

The midwives have all been very enthusiastic about the water births and are actually surprised that it has been such a positive experience:

- there are fewer women with muscle cramps in the legs;
- it gives great relief for those with pelvic pains;
- gives much mobility to everyone;
- there is less or no need to support the women physically when changing positions;
- the babies are more quiet and aware just after birth;
- the women feel more self confident;
- they are in charge of their situation, which results in a good experience of giving birth.

When preparing for this talk I asked the staff to identify any negative effects, but no one could think of any worth mentioning.

Introducing water births has been a positive challenge for the midwives and the other caregivers in our unit, giving increased joy in the work for everyone involved, including the doctors who all support our work.

Equipment

Finally, I would like to leave you with an impression of how we have arranged our delivery rooms to accommodate water births.

We have two delivery rooms, the photograph is of our largest room. The water tub is actually a large plastic container designed for industry. It holds 6-700 litres. For hygienic reasons, we use a clean liner and for filling the tub we use a disposable oxygen tube to prevent contamination of the water with bacteria from the ordinary hose pipe.

The tub is movable and is placed just above the drain. We have a waterproof sonic aid which is a very good investment.

Our most used remedy is an inflatable bathing ring, used for floating in the water. It gives excellent support to the woman's head and shoulders, and is perfect for relaxing between contractions. (It was bought in a toy store last summer for less than two pounds).

We can also recommend the large rubber balls (made for gymnastic exercises) as they are perfect for sitting by the tub - one for the partner, one for the midwife, so you will need two. They provide excellent working positions for the midwife, enables her to relax and keep a straight back, avoiding the twists common at bedside births.

The following is a list of the water birth equipment used in Fåborg:

- birth tub = plastic container
- plastic liner
- foam pipe insulation for edge of tub
- long veterinary gloves
- bath thermometer
- sieve for 'dirt' in the water
- foam mats for tub/kneeling on
- large rubber balls for sitting by the tub
- inflatable ring for floating in the water
- waterproof sonic aid.

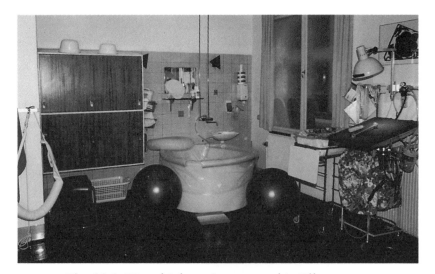

Fig. 20.1: Water birth equipment used in Fåborg

The cost of establishing a water birth facility has been approximately £500 per delivery room. With the use of warm water, lining, oxygen tube and gloves, estimated cost per delivery in water is a maximum of £3.00.

On the other hand, the use of other disposable materials has diminished as the use of water has increased.

As to our training, we have used our skills as midwives and have gained our experience bit by bit, bearing in mind that we are the ones who attend the delivering woman; we help the woman deliver her baby.

We have recently bought a third tub for use at home births, as we thought these women should have the same opportunities as those in the hospital. We are happy to attend home births.

Our tub can be borrowed for a token sum of £10.

Having water births can only be recommended. It is a cheap and uncomplicated way of offering a unique alternative for normal delivery, giving the midwives joy in their work, the women good experiences of birth and the babies a gentle entry into this world.

Footnote
Instructions for water birth
FÅBORG MATERNITY UNIT

According to our instructions, the aim of a water birth is especially the analgesia and relaxing effect a woman in labour attains by staying in the water while contracting and giving birth.

- In order to have a water birth, the woman must be healthy with a normal pregnancy and:

  - be at term (between 37 and 42 weeks of gestation)
  - be expecting a normal delivery with a baby in the vertex presentation
  - have clear liquor
  - be within 24 hours of ruptured membranes
  - have had no pethidine or Entonox
  - no signs of fetal distress

- The delivery must be supervised according to the usual procedures for a normal delivery on 'dry ground'.

- If necessary the woman in labour must lift her body out of the water - to hear the FHR and for vaginal examinations, but it can be done in the water.

- There should always be an adult person present, when a woman in labour is in the pool.

- Encourage lots of fluids.

- If ruptured membranes, check temperature. If showing a temperature the woman is not allowed in the water.

- The water temperature should be no more than 37C.

- The water should not reach above the woman's chest.

- Long gloves should be used for vaginal examinations and delivery.

- The woman in labour should be aware:

  - that the midwife may encourage her to feel how far the baby's head has come in the second stage.
  - that she has to stand up and deliver, if the baby's shoulders are not born after two contractions.
  - that she has to leave the pool for the third stage.
  - that she can leave the pool at any time if she wants to.

- The water birth should be registered in the birth register and in the mother's and baby's journal.

- The midwife is responsible for cleaning the tub after use.

Parity			Gestation			Orif. Start Water		
0 para	68	29.06%	37 week	1	0.43%	0 cm	0	0.00%
1 para	105	44.87%	38 week	13	5.56%	1 cm	1	0.43%
2 para	49	20.94%	39 week	26	11.11%	2 cm	2	0.85%
3 para	11	4.70%	40 week	61	26.07%	3 cm	25	10.69%
4 para	1	0.43%	41 week	55	23.50%	4 cm	29	12.39%
			42 week	36	15.38%	5 cm	49	20.94%
			>42 week	2	0.85%	6 cm	23	9.83%
			unreg.	40	17.09%	7 cm	25	10.68%
						8 cm	17	7.26%
						9 cm	7	2.99%
						10 cm	10	4.27%
						unreg.	46	19.66%
Total	234	100%	**Total**	234	100%	**Total**	234	100%

Time in Water			Perineal trauma			Weight (g)		
0 -15 mins	8	3.42%	none	81	34.62%	>2500	2	0.85%
15 mins-1hr	63	26.92%	labia	36	15.38%	2500-3000	26	11.11%
1-2 hrs	81	34.62%	gr.1	66	28.21%	3000-3500	84	35.90%
2-3 hrs	30	12.82%	gr.2	63	26.92%	3500-4000	90	38.46%
3-4 hrs	12	5.13%	gr.3	3	1.28%	4000-4500	20	8.55%
4-5 hrs	1	0.43%				4500-5000	9	3.85%
5-6 hrs	5	2.14%	epis	2	0.85%	<5000	1	0.43%
<6hrs	3	1.28%				unreg.	2	0.85%
unreg.	31	13.25%						
Total	234	100%				**Total**	234	100%

Apgar score				
	1 min		5 min	
0 points	0	0.00%	0	0.00%
1 points	0	0.00%	0	0.00%
2 points	0	0.00%	0	0.00%
3 points	0	0.00%	0	0.00%
4 points	0	0.00%	0	0.00%
5 points	1	0.43%	0	0.00%
6 points	2	0.85%	0	0.00%
7 points	8	3.42%	1	0.43%
8 points	17	7.26%	0	0.00%
9 points	99	42.31%	4	1.71%
10 points	107	45.73%	229	97.86%
Total	234	100%	234	100%

Third stage		
0-10 min	38	16.24%
10-30 min	94	40.17%
30 min - 1 hour	24	10.26%
more than 1 hour	52	2.14%
unreg	72	30.77%
ablatio	1	0.43%
Total	234	100%

Diverse		
shoulder	3	1.28%
PPH	5	2.14%
home	4	1.71%

Table 20.3: Water births in Fåborg from September 1993 to March 1995

Who can deliver in water?

Fåborg Maternity Unit offers a water birth to all women who have had a normal pregnancy and expect a normal delivery

Many prefer to be in the pool during first stage of labour because the water is pain relieving and gives much mobility.

If you don't want to get out of the tub when the second stage begins, then you can deliver in the water.

It is not dangerous for either the mother or the baby according to the facts from maternity units who practice water births both here and in the rest of the world.

The element the baby is born into resembles where it came from, and therefore it doesn't breathe before surfacing. Being born under water is a gentle entry into this world.

The delivery

The delivery takes place in a plastic tub which has a diameter of 1.30 m and a depth of about 65 cm. It contains about 6-700 litres.

The water is 37° and in order for the tub to be really clean, we use plastic liners for every delivery.

During delivery the midwife is at the side of the tub. As a water birth requires a more active effort on the woman's part, the midwife only assists with the last part of delivering the baby's head and shoulders and the lifting of the baby out of the water.

A woman in labour must however, be willing to allow the midwife to check FHR at any time precisely as would be done during delivery on 'dry ground'.

A woman in labour must also be prepared to get out of the tub if the midwife decides that it is irresponsible to continue the delivery in water. For example this could be:

Meconium stained liquor, unexpected bleeding, fetal distress, prolonged labour, if there is a need for medication, or because the midwife or the woman no longer feels safe with a water birth.

When the baby is born, mother and baby stay safely in the warm water for a short period and then are helped over to a bed for the third stage of labour.

The placenta is not delivered in the tub because the risk of contaminated water entering the empty uterus.

Until now more than 200 babies have been born in water at Fåborg Maternity Unit and every single delivery has been a very good experience for everyone involved.

If you want to know more about the use of water in labour and pain, please feel free to contact us.

Best wishes

The midwives in Fåborg

P.S. If you plan to have a home birth, you can borrow a water tub. Ask your midwife for further information.

Fig.20.2 : Guidelines for water birth

PART EIGHT

Water Birth –
The Way Forward

CHAPTER TWENTY ONE

Evaluating Immersion in Water: Issues to be Considered Regarding a Randomized Controlled Trial

Judy Bothamley is a midwife teacher currently studying full-time for a Masters in Midwifery with Thames Valley University. She is developing her role as a midwife researcher working on the Immersion in Water for Labour study with the Centre for Midwifery Practice, Queen Charlotte's Hospital, and also on Choices for Childbirth in a multi ethnic area for Brent and Harrow Health Agency.

Joanne Chadwick is a senior lecturer in Midwifery at Thames Valley University in London and teaches on both the MA and BSc programmes. She has recently completed an MSc in Health Education and has published several articles on midwifery related topics. Joanne is also a practising midwife and is currently involved in planning a randomized controlled trial to examine the use of immersion in water for labour and birth.

The use of water in labour and at birth is still controversial and further evaluation is clearly needed. It has been suggested that a large scale randomized controlled trial (RCT) is required, to evaluate reliably the benefits and hazards of immersion in water (McCandlish and Renfrew, 1993). But the planning of such a trial is fraught with difficulties encompassing both ethical and pragmatic problems. If properly planned and executed such an approach would facilitate control over variables, so aiming to avoid bias and provide a basis for the standard methods of statistical analysis, such as significance tests (Pocock, 1984).

Justification for a randomized controlled trial

In considering this approach, the investigator must take into account two main obligations to the client or trial participant. First, to safeguard individual rights and second, to facilitate research aimed at improving treatment and care (Lilford, 1995). The difficulty here is that only in an ideal world would there be no known differences between the treatments at the outset of the trial; ethically, therefore, all participants would be receiving appropriate treatment. In the real world the degree of equipoise is difficult to gauge, both collectively and individually. This consideration needs to be balanced against the knowledge that with non-randomized studies it is very difficult to obtain a reliable assessment of treatment efficacy (Pocock, 1984).

Planning a trial

Undertaking an RCT concerned with immersion in water constitutes an intellectual challenge with few clear-cut answers. Many areas require careful consideration and involve close collaboration with appropriate colleagues.

Initially a systematic review of the literature is required, which should have both a national and an international focus in order to facilitate the widest possible collection of data and opinion. The collecting together of interested clinicians and experienced researchers to discuss and give direction to the research questions is important from the outset in order to establish useful collaborative relationships. Following such a systematic review, the main issues of interest need to be identified. For immersion in water these might be safety, effectiveness in promoting pain relief, and client satisfaction. From these issues, a major research question can be defined - does immersion in water in labour and at birth reduce the need for pharmacological pain relief? Although this question then creates a basis for the trial, it also raises a host of problems that need to be answered.

Problems

There will be many confounding factors in a RCT of immersion in water for labour and at birth which include client parity, previous experience in labour, the stage of labour at randomization, the time spent in water and degree of ambivalence. A large multi-centred trial is perhaps the best way by which to achieve meaningful results whereby sufficient numbers of participants will negate the effects of confounding factors. Adequate funding, trial expertise and sound collaborative networks will be fundamental to the success of conducting a trial of this size.

In addition, the problem of assessing the cost and possible benefits of this approach must be considered. The cost of installing facilities for immersion in water, heating water and cleaning the pool after use, needs care and accuracy. Another component of this analysis needs to examine the cost of midwife time spent with women using water, compared with that of time spent with those who do not.

Participants

The most obvious problem of a RCT would be in recruiting sufficient women who are both ambivalent about pain relief and willing to be randomized. From preliminary studies carried out in Oxford and Sheffield in 1992, McCandlish and Renfrew (1993) suggested that more than 50 per cent of pregnant women might be prepared to participate in an RCT. It is hard to gauge whether a comparable number of women in 1996 will have the same view. Negative media coverage in 1993 might prove to have been significant. In addition, an increased availability and acceptance of water birth, plus a greater encouragement of choice in childbirth might have reduced the number of women who are ambivalent, rather than decided, as to their choice of pain relief. Cammu et al (1994) suggested that the increased availability of water immersion for labour would make the organisation of a large RCT very difficult. Once such discussion around recruitment to the trial has occurred, a woman (having been previously undecided) might develop a preference. Randomisation, therefore, might cause disappointment and so interfere with results. It is also important to realise that the degree of support given in labour must be uniform on both arms of the trial, otherwise outcomes would be strongly influenced by either the continued presence or absence of the midwife. Ideally, each participant would have attention solely from one midwife; however, in many busy maternity units this would present a problem.

Midwives

Midwives' attitudes about the use of water will inescapably affect the care they give to women, their interpretation and reporting of outcomes, and the information they give at the recruitment stage of the trial.

Different midwives will vary in the extent of their experience and levels of confidence. Nightingale (1994), in an article on water birth in practice, implies in her conclusion that as midwives became more experienced in conducting water birth, so safety improved. A large multi-centred trial would inevitably involve midwives who are relatively inexperienced in the conduct of deliveries in water. The Bristol Third Stage Trial was criticised for this very point, in that midwives were not experienced with the experimental treatment. Part of the preliminary work for such a trial must, therefore, involve establishing what constitutes adequate experience and education for midwives concerning water birth.

Analysis

A feature of a well designed RCT is that both groups are unaware of the treatment to which they are randomized. Inevitably, this is not possible for a water birth RCT; subjectivity is thereby introduced. For the purpose of analysis, the two randomized groups would need to be based upon the notion of 'intention to treat'. This raises the further question of how to analyse 'time spent in water' as individual women will spend different amounts of time in the water. Some may use water for a period of hours while others may only use it for a few minutes or not at all. The analysis will need to be designed with this constraint in mind.

A way forward

In noting the potential problems associated with designing a RCT for immersion in water, one wonders whether an alternative way forward would be to incorporate a 'preference' option within the RCT design. This would involve women either being randomized or joining a treatment group of their choice. This would mean that women's choices would not be compromised, and that some of the problems concerning degrees of ambivalence would be negated. The trial would need to be a large multi-centred trial with enough participants to demonstrate any differences between the groups. Qualitative data is also vital to explore such issues as the effect of trial participation for the women, and the experiences of the midwives involved. Finally, the results from any RCT also need to be considered alongside the ongoing National Audit conducted by the National Perinatal Epidemiology Unit, and the monitoring of adverse outcomes by the British Paediatric Association Surveillance Unit.

Note: Judy Bothamley and Joanne Chadwick did not present a paper at the International Water Birth Conference, but in view of the importance of carefully evaluating new technologies and procedures it was felt important to include a contribution on future randomized controlled trials in these proceedings.

References

Cammu, H., Clasen, K., Van Wettere, L., Dere, M. (1994). 'To bathe or not to bathe during the first stage of labour', *Acta Obstetrica Gynecol Scand,* 73, pp.468-472.

Lilford, R.J. (1995). 'Equipoise and the ethics of randomisation', *Journal of the Royal Society of Medicine,* 88, pp.552-559.

McCandlish, R., Renfrew, M. (1993). 'Immersion in water during labour and birth: the need for evaluation', *Birth,* 20(2), pp.79-85.

Nightingale, C. (1994). 'Waterbirth in practice', *Modern Midwife,* Vol.4, No.1, pp.15-19.

Pocock, S.J. (1984). *Clinical Trials: A Practical Approach,* Chicester: John Wiley and Sons.

CHAPTER TWENTY TWO

Water Birth – The Safety Issues

> **Yehudi Gordon** is an obstetrician and gynaecologist who has worked in three teaching hospitals in London and has a background of research into fetal well-being. Since 1979 he has defended parents' rights and has established water pools at the Garden Hospital. Yehudi is especially interested in creating a homelike atmosphere in hospital to encourage normal, natural birth. He is the author of many research papers and is co-author of *The Encyclopaedia of Pregnancy and Birth* and *Waterbirth*.

Humans evolved from the sea and within every person there is an internal sea. Eighty per cent of our bodies are composed of water and the rest consists of other elements and molecules. Unborn babies live in the watery world of the amniotic cavity. It is no wonder that pregnant women often have an affinity for water but many people are afraid of it and they are worried about the risk to the baby of drowning after birth in water. This paper addresses the safety of mother and baby when a birth pool is available for use.

Women who have a water birth are more satisfied with the experience than women who give birth on land; this was discussed by Faith Haddad during this conference. It follows that provided it is safe water birth is the preferred option for many women, in our hospital over 70 percent of women choose to labour in water and 25 to 30 percent of births occur in water.

Policies about birth in water

An International Survey of Maternity Units and Homebirth Practitioners was conducted by the author to ascertain the policies with regard to birthing in water. Telephone interviews were completed with 13 units and the findings are shown in Table 22.1 (shown overleaf).

Category	Excluded	Included
Gestation <36 weeks	11	2
Fetal growth retardation	2	11
Severe pre-eclampsia	12	1
Ruptured membranes	2	11
Meconium in amniotic fluid	2	11
Multiple pregnancy	12	1
Previous caesarean section	2	11

Table 22.1: Criteria for excluding women from birth in water

(Countries surveyed: Australia, Austria, Belgium, Denmark, France, Germany, Malta, South Africa, United Kingdom, USA).

The same survey revealed a number of rules about the use of the pool in labour (Table 22.2).

Rule	Followed	Not followed
Time limit in the pool	2	11
Minimum dilation on entering	3	10
Water temperature <37C	10	3
Intermittent fetal heart monitor	13	0
Cardiotocograph on admission	7	6
Analgesic in the pool	5	8
Vaginal examination in the pool	13	0

Table 22.2: Rules about the use of the pool in labour

The survey provides a useful set of guidelines, based on a combined experience of many thousands of water births, for practitioners setting out to use water for birth.

Trials on the use of water in labour or birth

Controlled trials

Trials which included control subjects and trialists have been both prospective randomized and retrospective non randomized (Table 22.3). In the randomized group there are only a small number of women who delivered in water, the rest used water for the first stage of labour so that larger numbers are needed to answer many interesting questions about the safety of birth in water. The information quoted is summarised from the 1993 paper by McCandlish and Renfrew (1993) and is derived from the Oxford database.

The authors concluded that in the randomized group one study showed that labour was longer in water, one showed less need for augmentation using syntocinon, and one showed fetal tachycardia without asphyxia. In the non randomized group one study showed faster cervical dilatation in water, three showed less need for analgesia and two showed less perineal trauma.

	Controls	Trialists
Randomized		
1st stage (3 trials)	242	246
2nd stage (1 trial)	29	25
Non randomized		
1st stage (2 trials)	151	177
2nd stage (3 trials)	375	342

Table 22.3: Trials on the use of water in labour or birth
Some of the trials quoted are ongoing.
British (National Perinatal Epidemiology Unit) Survey 1992-1993.

A total of 12,749 pregnancies were studied, water was used for labour alone by 8,255 women and there were 4,494 water births. The study did not include a control group of women who did not use water. There were 12 perinatal deaths described in the study, a perinatal mortality rate of 1.2 per thousand and the authors concluded that there was no evidence that the use of water conferred any additional risk to mother or baby. The authors also stated that more information was needed from prospective randomized trials. To assess events which occur infrequently large numbers of births are needed and multicentred trials must be used.

A new study is in progress, under the control of the British Paediatric Association Surveillance Unit, to collect data from questionnaires sent to the paediatric department of every hospital for a 12 month period during 1994-1995. The criteria for inclusion in the study are:

* labour or birth in water;
* perinatal death (stillbirth or death within 7 days) or
* admission to special care during the first 48 hours of life.

The analysis will compare adverse outcomes with data, derived from a low risk control group of women, obtained from regional data bases. This survey is expected to provide useful information about the nationwide incidence of neonatal complications associated with the use of water for labour and/or birth.

Safety issues

Maternal temperature

The temperature of the mother during labour may be an important factor in relation to the well-being of the baby. The fetus is entirely dependent on the mother for temperature control, with an equilibrium between the temperature of the blood in the fetal circulation in the placental vessels and the temperature of the blood in the maternal uterine blood vessels which supply the placenta.

A rise in temperature of the fetus increases the metabolic demands for oxygen and glucose, which may be in short supply in pregnancies complicated by placental insufficiency or hypoxia in labour. Two case reports of pregnancies complicated by intrapartum asphyxia have been published where the mothers used water for pain relief in labour but the births occurred on land (Rosevear et al, 1993). The authors speculated that the intrapartum hypoxia was related to the effect of a hot pool on the maternal and fetal temperature. The hypothesis is not proven, nevertheless the majority of units practising water birth now have a policy of recording and regulating the temperature of the water in the pool (Table 22.2). Prolonged immersion in the water is more likely to affect the maternal core temperature than a quick dip in the pool. The pool temperature is usually kept below 35°C during the first stage and below 37°C during the second stage of labour, whereas the maternal temperature is maintained at or below 37°C.

Perineal tears and episiotomy

The incidence of episiotomy among women delivering in water is much lower than birth on land and many midwives do not perform episiotomies in the pool. The episiotomy rate is usually under ten per cent when the baby is born in water. The rate of perineal trauma (lacerations and/or episiotomy) tends to be lower in women who deliver in water, the effect is greater in the first pregnancy (Burns and Greenish, 1993). Lacerations tend to be smaller with water birth and the incidence of second degree tears is lower (Table 22.4)

	Water birth n=117	Land birth n=207
Intact	44%	35%
1st degree tear	35%	25%
2nd degree tear	21%	35%
Episiotomy	0%	5%

Table 22.4: Perineal tears and episiotomy during spontaneous birth at St John and St Elizabeth Hospital 1994-1995

Delivery of the placenta

In a paper published in 1983 Michel Odent suggested the theoretical possibility of water entering the vagina and the uterine cavity as the placenta is born. He speculated that this could then lead to the absorption of water into the uterine veins draining the placental bed and cause a water embolus (Odent, 1983). This hypothesis is conjectural and to date there has not been a case of water embolus reported in the literature. The majority of midwives who attend water births support women staying in the pool during the third stage of labour to deliver the placenta providing that there is no clinical indication to leave the water e.g. excessive vaginal bleeding or feeling faint.

Protecting the midwife's back

There is a big advantage in having a pool which is permanently installed and plumbed in rather than a portable pool which may need to be moved or pumped to drain after use. A permanent pool is as easy to use as an ordinary bath.

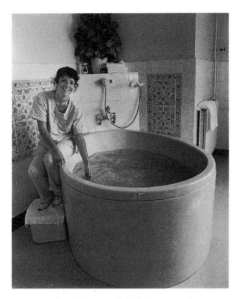

Fig. 22.1: A birthing pool

Modern birth pools usually provide a low stool which may be used as a seat for the midwife or as a footstool to assist the mother to enter or leave the pool. The majority of pools are installed at the same level as the floor of the birth room and this reduces the distance which the midwife has to bend during the birth.

The midwife needs to maintain a continuous state of awareness of her own posture when she is attending to the mother. It is safest to bend from the hips rather from the middle of the spine as the midwife reaches into the water to monitor the baby or to assist with the birth. This awareness is particularly important if there is a history of a previous back problem.

Shoulder dystocia

Shoulder dystocia is an obstetric emergency which every midwife fears and tries to avoid. Women at high risk of shoulder dystocia are encouraged to leave the pool in the second stage of labour before the birth, the list includes:

- A past history of shoulder dystocia
- A large baby (>4.0Kg)
- Prolonged labour, particularly a prolonged second stage

If an unexpected dystocia occurs the mother is helped out of the pool immediately by the birth attendants. A low stool for the woman to step onto is invaluable to ease the strain of moving after the baby's head has been delivered. The mother's movements as she leaves the pool are likely to help the baby's shoulders to enter the pelvic cavity and expedite the birth (Gibb, 1995; Macdonald and Stirk, 1995).

Midwifery units are expected to have a protocol for the management of shoulder dystocia and the different methods which are used to deliver the baby have recently been reviewed by Donald Gibb (1995). The mother cannot push with her maximum power in water but if she squats on the floor, supported by the birth attendants, then the downward pressure to assist the birth is greatest and the midwife is able to help by exerting gentle traction on the baby's head. If this is not sufficient additional pressure may be applied to the anterior shoulder of the baby by a birth attendant pressing on the supra pubic area, as the mother continues the supported squat. Squatting also allows the midwife to perform an episiotomy and to exert direct internal traction on the baby's shoulder to assist the delivery. The alternative to squatting is to use the hyper flexed position of the mother's hips while she lies on the bed which is the horizontal equivalent of squatting,

Infection

The risk of maternal infection is not increased when women use the pool during labour or for birth. Vaginal examinations are considered safe and are performed routinely while the mother is in the water (Table 22.2). Water is used for labour and birth after spontaneous rupture of the membranes (McCandlish and Renfrew, 1993).

Maternity units with a pool cleanse and sterilize the pool with an antiseptic solution every time it has been used. A small number of case reports have appeared in the literature describing postnatal infections in neonates, which have all responded to treatment (Rawal et al, 1994; George, 1990). None of the controlled trials have shown an increase in neonatal infection, (Table 22.3) nor was there an increased incidence found in the British National Perinatal Epidemiology Unit survey (see previously). If careful attention is paid to pool hygiene the neonatal infection risk is minimal.

Fetal hypoxia and water inhalation

Before birth the fetus breathes for about 40 per cent of the time and breathing is essential for growth of the fetal lung.

Breathing is inhibited by a number of mechanisms:

- Prostaglandin E2 - is a hormone produced in the placenta, the level rises before labour and the effect may continue during the labour and the birth.
- Warm temperature - if the pool water is kept at 37°C.
- Mild hypoxia - causes apnoea but severe hypoxia causes the fetus to gasp.
- Inhalation of fresh water - The entrance to the fetal larynx is lined with many chemoreceptors because the area serves both breathing and swallowing and it is essential for survival that fluid is not inhaled. During intrauterine life there is very little aspiration of amniotic fluid because lung liquid, with a low pH, is produced in the airway and it then flows out into the larynx to be swallowed. Amniotic fluid and lung fluid are isotonic (fluids which will mix without causing any disturbance) and both contain electrolytes whereas fresh water has few electrolytes and is hypotonic (a weaker solution) (Johnson, 1995).

Water in the larynx causes the diving response - apnoea, swallowing, arousal, bradycardia and hypertension. Blood flow is redistributed to the brain, heart and adrenal glands as part of the defence response. One or two drops of water are sufficient to trigger the diving response in the new-born baby and instead of inhaling the water it is swallowed.

The diving response is blunted by some drugs, e.g. atropine and beta blockers and these are not used in labour.

The diving response is also inhibited in severe, prolonged hypoxia. In mild hypoxia the fetus responds with apnoea but this changes when the hypoxia is severe and prolonged. A fetus who enters labour well nourished has a reserve of glycogen stores to provide energy, via anaerobic pathways, if hypoxia occurs. If there has been intra-uterine growth retardation the glycogen stores are depleted and if hypoxia occurs the fetus gasps earlier. The gasping response will override apnoea if mild hypoxia becomes severe and gasping is the mechanism involved in meconium aspiration in utero. Gasping is more dangerous after water birth than after birth on land because of the risk of inhalation of water.

All pregnancies are monitored routinely to detect fetal heart changes before severe hypoxia occurs. The midwife attending the birth will have noted antenatal or intrapartum clinical risk factors before the second stage of labour to aid the detection of intrapartum hypoxia prior to the birth. In Sweden a study of 120,000 new-born babies weighing less than 2.5Kg showed an incidence of a low Apgar score (0-3) of 8 per thousand (Kilander, 1992). Some of the low scores were not anticipated and two babies per thousand had an unforeseen and unanticipated Apgar score of 0-3 - these are the babies who may be at risk of gasping and inhalation at birth. A combination of clinical midwifery experience and skill combined with intrapartum monitoring and surveillance reduces the inhalation risk to a minimum.

Resuscitation of the new-born baby is a skill which every midwife needs to practice to the level of advanced neonatal resuscitation. A number of birth units have recently devolved the responsibility for resuscitation of term new-born infants from the neonatal paediatrician to the midwife with the paediatrician in a backup role (Raffles and Chandra, 1995). Training programs are available in the UK for midwives and obstetricians to acquire the advanced resuscitation skills, which include intubation and the administration of drugs, and continuous monitoring by the trainers ensure that every member of the team is updated and maintains regular practice of the techniques. In a number of birth units and on the training courses the trainers are nurses or midwives rather than doctors and the standards are set and maintained by the Resuscitation Council.

Birth in water is a relatively recent development in modern obstetric units and its introduction has been met with a mixed response from midwives, obstetricians and parents. The emotions range from intense enthusiasm to severe criticism of the use of water for labour and birth. Most of the critics have few objections about using water for pain relief in the first stage of labour, provided the temperature of the water is monitored and controlled; water is regarded as a harmless passing fad (Walker, 1994) Birth in the pool is a different matter and the critics are vociferous in predicting that water birth is hazardous for the baby, although there is no evidence in the literature to substantiate the predications. In common with all new techniques water birth certainly requires ongoing audit and evaluation as an increasing number of hospitals acquire pools. The results of the British paediatric Association survey, which are expected to be published later this year, will provide additional information, on a nationwide scale about the safety of water birth and a number of randomized controlled trials are in progress or are being planned. The enthusiasts are confident that water birth will continue to maintain the safety record which has emerged in the studies which have been conducted and analysed at this time.

References

Burns, E., Greenish, K. (1993). 'Pooling information', *Nursing Times,* Vol.89, pp.47-49.

George, R. (1990). 'Bacteria in birthing tubs'. *Nursing Times,* Vol. 86, p.14.

Gibb, D. (1995). 'Shoulder dystocia: The Obstetrics'. *Clinical Risk,* Vol.1, pp.49-54.

Johnson, P. (1995). 'Birth under water - to breathe or not to breathe'. Personal Communication.

Kilander, P. (1992). 'Methods of resuscitation in low Apgar score newborn infants'. *Acta Paediatrica,* Vol.8, pp.739-745.

McCandlish, R., Renfrew, M. (1993). 'Immersion in water during labour and birth: the need for evaluations'. *Birth,* Vol.20, pp.79-85.

Macdonald, S., Stirk, F.D. (1995). 'Shoulder dystocia: Midwives' role'. *Clinical Risk,* Vol.1, pp.61-65.

Odent, M. (1983). 'Birth under water', *The Lancet,* Vol.2, pp.1476-1477.

Raffles, A., Chandra, C. (1995). *Guidelines for resuscitation in term infants are safe and effective.* In press.

Rawal, J., Shah, A., Stirk, F., Mehtar, S. (1994). 'Water birth and infection in babies'. *British Medical Journal,* Vol.309, p.511.

Rosevear, S.K., Fox, R., Marlow, N., Stirrat, G.M. (1993). 'Birth pools and the fetus'. *The Lancet.* Vol.342, pp.1048-1477.

Walker, J.J. (1994). 'Birth underwater: sink or swim'. *British Journal of Obstetrics and Gynaecology,* Vol.101, pp.467-468.

CHAPTER TWENTY THREE

Surviving the Onslaught of the Uninformed

> **Lesley Page** is the Queen Charlotte's Professor of Midwifery Practice and the only practising midwife member of the English National Board. She served on the Expert Maternity Group which wrote the government policy document on the maternity services, *Changing Childbirth*. She has supported women through both home births and water births. She lectures widely in the UK and overseas, is author of many papers, and is editor of *Effective Group Practice in Midwifery: Working with Women*. (Blackwell Science, 1995).

This weekend has been an amazing event. A gathering of clinicians, scientists, epidemiologists, activists, all inspired by the need to explore further the potent effect of this new, and mind altering, approach to birth in water. We are united by the same mission. To find better ways of birth, birth which is healthy and wholesome. Birth which retains and reflects the poetry. To honour the miracle of the birth of the new born into the world, and to help as the woman gives birth to herself as mother.

Each one of you will have known the loneliness of trying something new. But each one of you will have experienced the sense of rightness of finding a better way. You will go away knowing that you are not alone, and there are many sharing the same aspirations and the same work. We are leaving with a far deeper understanding of clinical standards, of the scientific basis and of the outcomes. This knowledge in itself will help you survive the onslaught of the uninformed. But this knowledge will not be enough in itself. You will also require political skills and courage.

Many in today's world are uninformed (Page and Kitzinger, 1995). Far too many people today assume that more technology has improved the quality and safety of birth.

Far too few people today question the effects of technology on birth. Far too few know how many women and babies are actually harmed by technology. That ignorance has become a major problem. A well known obstetrician recently made the headlines saying 'they are all mad' in regard to the question of water birth. I wonder what he thinks madness is? Abdominal incision? In many parts of the world, particularly North America, a quarter of the population give birth to their babies through an abdominal incision. The real insanity lies in accepting that. Britain has retained a relative degree of sanity. But even here caesarean sections are on the rise. Even here the majority of women receive continuous electronic fetal monitoring in their labour. And even here large numbers of women feel they need an epidural as the only way to cope with the pain of labour.

Despite a huge and powerful onslaught from various obstetricians (Jenkins and Tyler, 1994), and even some midwives, the belief in the value of water birth has persisted. Thousands of women ignore the warnings: more and more women still use immersion in water for labour and the birth of their babies.

Water birth is a symbol of natural, joyful birth. The birthing pool offers a natural way for women to use the therapeutic effects of water, it provides an oasis of privacy for their own attendant midwife away from the usual atmosphere of the delivery suite: it respects the social dimension of this great event in their lives.

Too many professionals have far too blinkered a perspective; they measure nothing but broad figures of maternal and infant mortality. These figures actually vindicate water birth as safer on strictly medical criteria. But we must also look at much wider questions: how can we best provide women with a rich and safe experience of labour and birth when they decide to use a pool?

So, we require wide exploratory studies of women's and midwives' experiences. What does the use of water in birth have in common with other, traditional approaches to midwifery care - approaches which have been nearly eradicated over the last 20 years in the industrialized world? They have in common the value we feel in human presence and touch, comforting words, calm atmosphere and an ability to celebrate this momentous event of human life. Because we are, pardon the pun, swimming against the mainstream, we will require more studies in a quantitative mode to evaluate outcomes, so that we can provide women with information to help them make the most appropriate decisions for them (McCandlish and Renfrew, 1993).

Our study should also explore standards for care to provide the greatest degree of protection possible for families who choose this approach to labour and birth. From the quantitative to the qualitative our thinking will require adjustments. For example, using water for labour is an attempt to help women cope with the pain rather than numbing them completely, as with an epidural. Water helps women cope with the pain of labour and possibly enhances those passions and deep emotions which are an integral part of healthy birth.

Importantly, when we look at the issue of safety and physical outcomes in water labour and water birth, we should compare this treatment with other treatments which are commonly accepted in the medical domain. For example, epidural anaesthesia which has been accepted as a natural form of care while immersion in water has been regarded as unnatural.

We already have, as a consequence of this important conference, the beginnings of answers to some of our questions.

We have discovered that midwives require different skills and approaches in the care of women who are immersed in water for labour. Trials and studies of water birth have indicated that the operative delivery rate may be reduced by the use of water. Although retrospective studies should be interpreted with caution, we have an indication that immersion in water for labour and birth may be as safe, if not safer, for a low risk population than other forms of care. We have heard the description of the intensity of experience when parents have used this approach to the birth of their babies.

The studies presented here provide an amalgamation of a large amount of experience. This conference is the beginning of a world wide collaboration between those committed to finding alternative ways of helping women give birth to their babies, alternative ways which we hope will become mainstream as we move away from technical, medical, surgical, anaesthetized birth.

At the Centre for Midwifery Practice in Queen Charlotte's and Hammersmith and Thames Valley University, we shall be co-ordinating a series of studies and working with others to share findings so that we may continue to answer questions about comparative safety, and continue to explore the experiences of women, doctors and midwives and the effect of this approach to birth which offers a way of helping women and their families regain power, personal and physical integrity, and family integrity around the time of birth. Water birth is both a potent symbol of fundamentally different way of birth, and a real practical alternative which may help us restore and enrich birth as a social and spiritual event.

References

Jenkins, R., Tyler, S. (1994). 'Water births give a bad press' (correspondence) *British Medical Journal*, 308, p.920.

McCandlish, R., Renfrew, M. (1993). 'Immersion in water during labour and birth. The need for evaluation' *Birth*, 20, pp.79-85.

Page, L., Kitzinger, S. (1995). 'A midwifery perspective on the use of water in labour and birth' *Midwifery*, 22 January, pp.22-26.

Water Birth Practice

We are collecting information on labour in water and water birth from around the world and keeping a register of information.

If you work in a hospital, birth centre, or home birth practice in which water is offered for labour and/or birth, we should welcome any information that you can let us have. Please write to the address given below for a questionnaire.

The Centre for Midwifery Practice,
Wolfson School of Health Sciences
Thames Valley University,
32-38 Uxbridge Road,
London W5 2BJ.